FEB 1 9 2019

D0804268

"Dave Meurer's latest book, *New Every Day: Navigating Alzheimer's with Grace and Compassion*, is a heartfelt and helpful guide to any family who has been touched by the long and painful journey of Alzheimer's. Written in Dave's signature style, this book delivers, and it takes some of the mystery out of this disease while giving hope, compassion, and a whole lot of grace to those on the front lines."

**Martha Bolton**, Emmy-nominated former staff writer for Bob Hope and author of over eighty books, including *Josiah for President* and *The Home Game*

"In a word, this book is fantastic! Dave has just the right balance of lighthearted humor when permissible, insight when needed, and valuable information throughout—all presented with charm and practicality. I loved it!"

**Marilyn Meberg**, author and speaker

"Dealing with a loved one who has Alzheimer's disease can be stressful and heartbreaking. You need support from someone who has been there. This book is like sitting down with a good friend, swapping stories, having a good cry, but also laughing together at some of your shared experiences. As a therapist, I highly recommend it. Laughter truly is good for the soul."

**Timothy R. Holler**, EdD, LPC-MHSP, cofounder, Sage Hill Counseling, Memphis, TN

"I found *New Every Day* to be both informative and entertaining. I appreciated the information on Alzheimer's/dementia issues and on all the issues involved in caring for loved ones. It was helpful to read about others' similar issues and how they handled them. Dave's book also showed that

FEB 18 2019

it is helpful to keep a good sense of humor and how to do that respectfully."

**Margaret Fielding,** registered nurse and caregiver

"It's obvious that Dave has truly experienced a family member with Alzheimer's. I'm impressed that he took it upon himself to learn everything he could about his mother-in-law's disease. His sense of humor along with his knowledge of the process is refreshing. I hope many families affected by Alzheimer's have the chance to read this!"

**Elizabeth M. Amlin,** community relations director
at Sundial Assisted Living

# New Every Day

# New Every Day

## NAVIGATING ALZHEIMER'S

### WITH GRACE AND COMPASSION

# DAVE MEURER

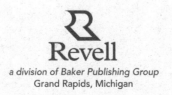

Revell

a division of Baker Publishing Group
Grand Rapids, Michigan

© 2018 by Dave Meurer

Published by Revell
a division of Baker Publishing Group
PO Box 6287, Grand Rapids, MI 49516-6287
www.revellbooks.com

Printed in the United States of America

All rights reserved. No part of this publication may be reproduced, stored in a retrieval system, or transmitted in any form or by any means—for example, electronic, photocopy, recording—without the prior written permission of the publisher. The only exception is brief quotations in printed reviews.

Library of Congress Cataloging-in-Publication Data
Names: Meurer, Dave, 1958– author.
Title: New every day : navigating Alzheimer's with grace and compassion / Dave Meurer.
Description: Grand Rapids, MI : Revell, a division of Baker Publishing Group, [2018] | Includes bibliographical references and index.
Identifiers: LCCN 2018020851 | ISBN 9780800734756 (pbk. : alk. paper)
Subjects: LCSH: Alzheimer's disease—Religious aspects. | Alzheimer's disease—Patients—Home care. | Alzheimer's disease—Patients—Family relationships.
Classification: LCC RC523 .M48 2018 | DDC 616.8/311—dc23
LC record available at https://lccn.loc.gov/2018020851

Unless otherwise indicated, Scripture quotations are from the Holy Bible, New International Version®. NIV®. Copyright © 1973, 1978, 1984, 2011 by Biblica, Inc.™ Used by permission of Zondervan. All rights reserved worldwide. www.zondervan.com

Scripture quotations labeled KJV are from the King James Version of the Bible.

Scripture quotations labeled NASB are from the New American Standard Bible®, copyright © 1960, 1962, 1963, 1968, 1971, 1972, 1973, 1975, 1977, 1995 by The Lockman Foundation. Used by permission. (www.Lockman.org)

This publication is intended to provide helpful and informative material on the subjects addressed. Readers should consult their personal health professionals before adopting any of the suggestions in this book or drawing inferences from it. The author and publisher expressly disclaim responsibility for any adverse effects arising from the use or application of the information contained in this book.

18   19   20   21   22   23   24        7   6   5   4   3   2   1

In keeping with biblical principles of creation stewardship, Baker Publishing Group advocates the responsible use of our natural resources. As a member of the Green Press Initiative, our company uses recycled paper when possible. The text paper of this book is composed in part of post-consumer waste.

To my amazing wife, Dale,
who has risen to each challenge
with grace and compassion.

# CONTENTS

# ACKNOWLEDGMENTS

I need to give a shout-out here to a few folks who played a key role in this book.

Several cubic yards of gratitude go to my editor, Lonnie Hull DuPont, who believed that a humor writer could take on a serious subject and not make a hot mess of it. Thank you for believing in this project, and for the very gentle edits.

I thank Peggy Whitten for her insights, for letting me quote her liberally, and for just being an all-around awesome person. The world does not know what you did for your mom, but God certainly does. And Greg Whitten has been the very model of a supportive spouse. You two really are a dynamic duo, only without the superhero outfits.

Kudos to Steve Laube, my agent, who has been there from the beginning of my writing career. Steve was my first cheerleader, but without the pom-poms and actual cheers, much less the acrobatic tricks.

Last, and by no means least, I want everyone to know that my sons Mark and Brad have been truly wonderful to their grandmother.

## ONE

# Sweet Little Lies

I find myself making the most outrageously misleading statements these days. I tried at first to avoid outright falsehoods, out of deference to one of the Ten Commandments, but quickly realized that *misleading* and *flat-out lies* are pretty much two sides of the same coin. Any reasonable jury would convict me of flagrant and deliberate deceit. And then they would give me a standing ovation as I accept my Oscar for Best Actor.

My creative misuse of the English language spares me the heartbreaking task of, once again, informing my eighty-six-year-old mother-in-law, Karin, that her husband has been deceased for years. And my trickery is precisely what the doctor ordered.

Karin (pronounced like "put the *car in* the garage") and I regularly have these kinds of conversations:

Karin: "I haven't seen Gene all morning. Do you know where he is?"

Me: "Well, you know those truck drivers. It seems like they're always on the road." (Attempt to dodge the question.)

Karin: "Is he in Oregon?"

Me: "He's picking up a load as we speak." (Massive whopper.)

She breathes a sigh of relief.

Karin: "I feel so much better. I was worried when he wasn't at breakfast."

Me: "He had to leave early. He said he hopes you have a nice day."

If I were Pinocchio, my nose would be in an entirely different solar system by now.

Welcome to the wild and woozy world of Alzheimer's disease, a slow but inexorable attack on the brain that creates massive confusion, memory loss, and increasingly diminished capacity to carry out the functions of daily life. Anything you said yesterday, or even five minutes ago, can be startling news.

Karin: "Why do I have this cast on my arm?"

Me: "You took a fall last week and fractured your wrist."

Karin: "Well, this is the first I've heard of it! Somebody should have told me about it!"

Me: "Sorry about that. We'll try to do a better job of communicating."

Karin: "I should hope so!"

We have now had that conversation dozens of times. For Karin, it is new every day.

But the person with Alzheimer's disease isn't the only one who is going to be off-kilter. Family and friends find themselves scrambling to come up with some kind of appropriate and calming reply to a series of decidedly peculiar comments, such as this exchange:

Karin: "There are six children living in my bathroom, and they need to go home."

Me: "Those rascals. I'll call their parents to pick them up." (Attempt to relieve her concern.)

Karin: "I don't know how they keep getting in."

Me: "Say, you are looking lovely today! I see you're wearing your favorite blouse." (Attempt to redirect her to a new subject.)

Karin: "I've never worn this before."

Me: "Ah. Yes. My mistake." (Never argue with someone who has Alzheimer's.)

Karin: "I've been camping in the wilderness for weeks!"

Me: "That must have been quite an adventure! Tell me more!" (Just roll with it.)

The World Health Organization estimates that, worldwide, roughly fifty million people have dementia, and that Alzheimer's disease constitutes 60 to 70 percent of cases. About five million of those cases are in the United States.[1]

One of those cases is Karin.

And, since you are reading this, it is likely the disease has taken hold in the life of someone you love.

I'm so sorry. I know what you are going through.

No one plans to have Alzheimer's disease crash into the life of a loved one any more than someone plans on being involved in a train wreck. But a problem never asks you if it is a convenient time to barge in the door.

"Not ready for a crisis? No worries. I'm flexible. Tuesday work for you? No? How about next week? I'm wide open at

11:00 a.m. on Friday. I may be a disaster, but I'm reasonable. Let's make this a win-win."

Doesn't happen that way.

Alzheimer's disease is one of those tragic events that elbows into your life, hurts someone you love, breaks your heart, bewilders your mind, disrupts your plans, impacts your finances, and consumes enormous amounts of time and emotional energy.

You need to sit down with a friend who is in the same boat, commiserate, share what has and hasn't worked, have a good cry, but also—importantly—have a good laugh at some of your mutual experiences. You need some joy on this hard slog of a journey. You can't go it alone. You need to be connected with someone who knows exactly what you are talking about when you shake your head and explain how you keep finding potato chips in Dad's underwear drawer.

Maybe I can play the role of a friend like that. (You still need to find someone who can actually take you out for coffee and a massive slice of coconut cream pie, but maybe I can pinch-hit for a bit.)

When I say you need to laugh, let me make it clear that we aren't laughing at our loved one or making light of the disease. But the situation you're in has the potential to drag you into a dark cave. I have read all kinds of books and articles on Alzheimer's disease, and while they have been informative and helpful, they are generally dry and, honestly, kind of depressing. I believe we need some laughter as we make our way down this long and painful road. And when something happens that makes you laugh, it's healthy to enjoy the moment.

Karin: "People keep saying I have that thing. What is it they say I have?"

Me: "Memory loss."

Karin: "Well, I don't!"

As is so often the case, the disease had been slowly unfolding for years. Karin had been mentally slipping for quite some time, but she was still living on her own. Cooking. Dressing herself. Visiting with other residents in the Happy Cedars Community for Dynamic Seniors (not the real name of the joint, but something equally excessive cooked up by marketing people with too much time on their hands).

My wife, Dale, and I visited Karin often, and thus began seeing the signs that her condition was worsening. Perishable groceries stored in the cupboard instead of the refrigerator. Her inability to operate the television remote control. The repeated surprise that Ronald Reagan wasn't still president, let alone not still breathing.

We decided to bring her to our home for the weekend to keep an eye on her and take her to the doctor the following Monday.

It was a bit after two o'clock in the morning when we had the rather arresting experience of having a police officer stand in our bedroom and shine his flashlight in our faces while explaining that he was responding to a 911 call.

"There mushed be some kinder mistake," I mumbled, blinking.

"Well, there is a confused elderly woman in your living room," he replied.

Ah. Yes.

My wife and I threw on our robes and joined the officer in the front room.

"Ma'am, do you know these folks?"

"Yes. That is my daughter and that is the man who drives the big brown van. But I have never been in this place before, and my husband is missing. So I called 911."

("Man who drives the big brown van?" I drive a Chrysler 300.)

I was punchy, disconcerted, and completely out of my element, so I stupidly replied, "Karin, you have been to our house a thousand times. And Gene passed away two years ago."

She looked utterly stunned.

"Well, this is the first I've heard of it," she replied softly.

I have learned a great deal since that ordeal, both by reading voraciously and availing myself of the wisdom of the professionals who are helping us navigate Alzheimer's disease.

"Enter her world, and don't try to correct her misperceptions," is one of the best pieces of advice I have received.

If she believes she spoke with her parents on the phone an hour ago, we now say, "I hope you had a good conversation." If she tells Dale she is working the evening shift at the hospital, my wife tells her what a valued employee she is. If she tells me she flew to Europe last night and asks me how they managed to get her back in time for breakfast, I simply ask, "Isn't it amazing what they can do these days?" And then I point out how beautiful the roses are.

With Alzheimer's or another type of dementia, sometimes the best you can do is provide peace in the moment. Often we find we can also bring joy. The standard biblical conventions about speaking the truth don't apply when you are dealing with someone with this disease. What good comes from making a loved one relive the loss of a spouse or parents when she is under the happy illusion that everyone she has ever loved is alive and well? Why feel the need to correct her if she says she spent the morning milking the cows? Just thank her for being such a great help on the farm.

So I thank the Academy for this Oscar, which I am happy to share with my wife for her supporting role in the zany comedy titled, *Of* Course *We Didn't Hide the Car Keys*.

# TWO

# Driven to Distraction

I *adore* the department of motor vehicles. Truly. While I dislike the long lines, the forms, the fees, the taxes, the interminable delays, and the implied message that all this is somehow necessary for me to simply drive from point A to point B, I am smitten with the DMV because they are the ones who took my mother-in-law off the road. I want to give them a collective kiss on their bureaucratic lips.

There are a hundred different telltale signs that a loved one is losing the capacity to drive. One of the first, subtle signs I witnessed was when Karin roared down our driveway, swerved to the side of our house, and skidded to a gravel-spewing stop a quarter inch from our gas meter. I nearly committed a hygienic impropriety.

Karin smiled as she ambled from the car, blissfully un-aware that she had come a few millimeters from detonating our house.

Tragically, what is becoming more and more obvious to you is often not at all obvious to the senior citizen who prizes her independence and still holds a license to operate what has essentially become a two-thousand-pound portable wrecking device. A license to drive represents freedom and independence, and if you even hint at taking it away, you can expect the kind of fierce resistance Napoleon encountered at Waterloo—only with more yelling involved and no French accents. You're going to need reinforcements.

I suggest a family intervention where you gently but frankly express concern about whether your loved one is having trouble driving. Sometimes this goes well, and the senior agrees to hand over the keys. I use the word *sometimes* in the same sense in which I note that *sometimes* Halley's comet streaks by the earth, or *sometimes* you win the lottery and have enough disposable income to purchase Jamaica. More commonly, the reaction is akin to asking a mother bear if you can keep one of her cubs. You might be able to regain some of your hearing a few hours after the roar stops ringing in your ears.

But this is where the wonderful and eminently smoochable people at the DMV come in. They let you rat someone out, but allow you to shroud your identity like you're in the witness protection program, and you just spilled the beans on Guido the Gun.

I made an appointment and told the clerk that my mother-in-law was getting lost, cruising through town for hours in search of stores she had been to hundreds of times, and often only vaguely aware of why she got behind the wheel in the first place.

She also blew through a red light at the absolutely worst intersection in town, for which she received a $450 ticket courtesy of the automated traffic cameras that record such events in case the accused wishes to argue the infraction.

And boy, did she want to argue.

"The city workers moved all the lights so they are much higher and almost impossible to see. I have never driven drunk in my entire life! I worked for the Salvation Army!" she fumed.

"Karin, no one is accusing you of drunk driving," I replied. "But that was extremely dangerous, and it could have seriously hurt or even killed you or someone else."

"That's why they shouldn't have moved the lights!" she exclaimed. "Besides, if they allow drunks on the road, then they should definitely allow me."

"Well, that's certainly one way to look at it."

I told her I would double check the intersection since I drive through it every day. Upon meticulous review of the scene, it was clear that the only thing that had changed were the various synapses and firing mechanisms in her brain that allowed her to recall, with crystal clarity, her first bicycle, but not what she had for dinner last night.

And thus came the notice in the mail.

The DMV people, all of whom richly deserve raises, official commendations, and all-expense paid trips to Paris, told her that she must make an appointment with her doctor and take a standardized test. This test included rigorous questions, such as "What year is this?"

Karin missed the correct answer by an entire decade. She also flamed out on most of the other questions.

"What is your address?"

"Oregon."

"What country are you in?"

"California."

"What month is this?"

"Easter."

The doctor also tested short- and long-term memory, attention span, concentration, and language skills.

"Karin, I'm going to say three objects and I want you to repeat them back to me in a moment; table, chair, plate. But first, count backward from one hundred, by fives."

"100, 90, 80, 70, 80, 90, 100."

"Thank you. Now repeat the three words I gave you a bit ago."

(Blank stare.)

She offered a couple of correct answers here and there, but her overall score was a spectacular failure. She was given a driving test—let's just say that the outcome was less than stellar, and the DMV ride-along observer is probably still not sleeping at night.

The results were duly reported to the DMV hierarchy, who informed Karin that her right to drive was hereby revoked. However, they gave her the right to appeal. But doing so would first require months of visits to a neuropsychiatrist, a battery of memory exercises, and dozens of tests. The entire exercise was just a massive, even ludicrous, waste of everyone's time. So of course, Karin insisted on it.

Dale tried to gently suggest that her mom just accept the results of the test, and assured Karin she could still get around. "I'll be your chauffer! We can have even more time together. How about if I take you shopping whenever you want to go?"

Karin had that same steely look in her eye that General Douglas MacArthur had when he announced that he would return. "I am *not* a drunk driver, and I *am* going to drive again!"

This meant scores of hours that Dale had to sit in a waiting room while her mom valiantly attempted to repeat simple phrases like "carrots, peas, and radishes" two minutes after memorizing them. After several months of this, Dale overheard Karin tell a friend, "I don't know why my daughter insists that I take these memory classes. They are a waste of time and money. But she is just so *bossy!*"

Let's just say Dale did not find this nearly as amusing as I did.

# THREE

# The Non-Chapter Note

Random note from Dave: This book isn't in any kind of chronological or logical order. I wrote stuff based on what was happening or what popped into my head at the moment, and figured I would organize the chapters later. Well, it is now later, and I still haven't changed the order. I have inserted this little note at the last minute before the book goes to press.

I have fussed around with stuff for a bit and puzzled over it, but I couldn't decide whether to begin at the beginning, or start with a robust examination of the disease, or put the most interesting material first.

In the end, I couldn't decide how to organize it. I finally decided that it didn't really matter. You're going to eventually plow through it all anyway, unless I haven't done my job. It is a crime to bore readers, and I don't want to be guilty of doing that.

So sometimes, later in the book, you will read about Karin in the early stages when the previous section discussed her life in the later stages. You will read about her living independently, after I already revealed in the first chapter that she is now in assisted living. The narrative disorder might make you scratch your head because it doesn't seem to make sense. Good. It is excellent training for life with Alzheimer's.

You will also find that some chapters are kind of short and some are quite long and completely inconsistent. (More good training.) Just adapt. And cut me some slack, because this illness keeps us hopping. Sometimes I barely have time to use the restroom. Those Depends are looking like an attractive option.

Thank you for your understanding.

# FOUR

# The Runaway

Evelyn was making a run for it.

Well, maybe it wasn't so much a *run* as it was a very slow mosey toward the front door of Festive Acres Senior Assisted Living.

Okay, I changed the name of the place, but it was called something kind of like that. All of those assisted-living homes name themselves something chipper and upbeat like Convivial Commons or Restful Roughage, but the name is for the family and not the residents. By the time you're in one of those places, you aren't really focused on what it's called. The home could have been called IHOP or Sears, and I don't think Evelyn would have known or cared. She just had a vague sense that she belonged somewhere else, and so she called out, "Well, I'll be leaving now!" and shuffled toward the front door.

I was there to witness what happened next because Karin also resides at Festive Acres, so Dale and I are often there for visits. And what we saw next wasn't an argument or a call to the police or a staff member tackling an octogenarian before she wandered out the front door. What happened was the deft response of a young lady named Kayla.

"Okay, Evelyn. Bye-bye."

Evelyn stepped toward the door.

"Oh, Evelyn, before you go—can you help me with something?" Kayla called from down the hall.

"Sure," replied Evelyn. And by the time she was down the hall, she had forgotten about leaving.

Kayla does not simply distract the residents. She engages with them, listens to their stories (over and over and over), and truly loves them. And it is beautiful to see in action.

It is hard to outrun the gift of mercy.

But next to mercy, redirection is your best friend when dealing with dementia. When Karin asks, "When am I going home?" we say, "Soon." Or, "Later." Or whatever we think might work based on her level of confusion that day. We don't say, "This is your new home," because that often produces confusion and an argument. (It works for other people, but not for her.)

Occasionally I will ask her if she trusts Doctor Arai (her lifelong physician). She always says yes. So I will reply, "He wants you to stay here tonight."

Nine times out of ten, she won't argue.

But there is no formula here. The redirections you employ could be unique to you and your loved one based on how well anything works on a given day. But here is what doesn't work—arguing. Telling the dementia sufferer he is wrong. Getting exasperated. Asking, "Don't you remember . . . ?"

Of *course* he doesn't remember! He's not being obstinate, or obtuse, or arguing for the sake of arguing. He has a progressive disease that has not only attacked his ability to remember events, but also befuddles his mind when he tries to do simple tasks like button his shirt or tie his shoes.

A person with neurocognitive disorder does not eat spaghetti with her hands because she lacks manners. She simply can't recall how to use a fork at that moment or thinks she is looking at finger food or because of any number of other reasons. And your reaction can make life either easier or more difficult. You get to be the one who adapts, because she cannot.

The Bible tells us that "Love is patient, love is kind . . ." (1 Cor. 13:4 NASB).

Love also learns to change the subject when it needs to.

"Let's have some lemon cake!" works way better than an argument.

# FIVE

# This Is Not Normal

Karin: "Should I introduce you as my niece?"

Dale: "Well, more like your daughter."

Karin (laughing): "That's right. How silly of me."

That conversation took place a few years ago when, sometimes, a clarification would actually help Karin understand reality. These days, Dale just rolls with however her mom views her.

This is not just a matter of old age.

A bit of memory loss can be normal as we get older, but Alzheimer's and other neurocognitive disorders aren't a normal part of aging. It is one thing to pause for a moment to grasp for a familiar word—it is another thing entirely to believe you are living in your childhood home three hundred miles away, your daughter is your niece (or, depending on the day, your mother), or that your deceased spouse just waved to you from the kitchen window. Profound mental confusion is a disease, not an inexorable part of aging. Most of us have met folks in their eighties who are razor-sharp mentally and living independently. *That* is normal. Having this conversation is not normal:

Karin (staring at her lunch): "What is *that*?"

Dale: "That's a salad, Mom."

Karin: "Well, I've never had one of those before and I am *certainly* not going to start now!"

Dale: "That's okay. We'll get you something else."

Although I tend to switch back and forth when using the words *dementia* and *Alzheimer's*, I should clarify that these are related, but not interchangeable, terms. *Dementia* is not the name of a disease, but rather an umbrella term that covers symptoms that impact memory, performance of routine activities of daily life, the ability to communicate, and the capacity to process information.

The National Institute of Neurological Disorders and Stroke (NINDS) explains that

> Alzheimer's disease (AD) is an age-related, non-reversible brain disorder that develops over a period of years. Initially, people experience memory loss and confusion, which may be mistaken for the kinds of memory changes that are sometimes associated with normal aging. However, the symptoms of AD gradually lead to behavior and personality changes, a decline in cognitive abilities such as decision-making and language skills, and problems recognizing family and friends. AD ultimately leads to a severe loss of mental function. These losses are related to the worsening breakdown of the connections between certain neurons in the brain and their eventual death. AD is one of a group of disorders called dementias that are characterized by cognitive and behavioral problems.[1]

"Cognitive and behavioral problems" is a fancy way of saying that Dad might flush his dentures down the toilet. Mom might misplace her jewelry and accuse you of stealing it. Grandma can mistake the recliner for the toilet.

The NINDS notes that Alzheimer's disease is the most common cause of dementia afflicting people who are sixty-five and older. It has causes that differ from, say, vascular dementia (generally considered the second most common form of dementia) and dementia with Lewy bodies (generally considered the third most common kind of dementia). But there is also frontotemporal dementia, Parkinson's disease dementia, Posterior Cortical Atrophy, and a handful of other variants.[2]

This can kind of seem like differentiating between saying "potato" or "po-tah-toe," because so many of the symptoms overlap. And though the causes are different, and each form of dementia may attack the brain from different angles, they all result in a progressively debilitating condition that affects memory, thought, and ability to function normally on a day-to-day basis. But I want you to know that there are various permutations of neurocognitive disorders, because it can be confusing to hear your doctor discuss "Lewy body dementia" (which often includes the kind of symptoms you see in Parkinson's disease) when you are under the impression that Alzheimer's is the only cause of dementia.[3]

(I should also note that some neurocognitive conditions hit very hard and very fast, with all the subtlety of General Patton's Third Army rolling through France. Researchers call these "rapidly progressive dementias" or RPDs.[4] I think of them as "rocket propelled dementias." The symptoms will be sudden and dramatic and are cause for burning rubber down to the hospital emergency room. But RPDs are not the norm for most dementias, and the underlying condition may respond to timely intervention. If you see it, treat it like the medical emergency it is.)

There is also the regrettable reality of "mixed dementia," a situation in which the particular markers of more than one type of dementia are present simultaneously. One of Karin's caregivers believes Karin had a non-Alzheimer's condition (vascular dementia) early on, because she could recall very specific details of a conversation she had with him nine months earlier. It was the kind of thing he didn't usually observe in his Alzheimer's patients. But as time wore on, Karin's treating doctors thought she clearly demonstrated the markers for Alzheimer's disease. She likely has more than one kind of dementia.

This is not an easy diagnosis to make, but the mixed dementia condition is very real. But again, the fundamental fact is that all of the irreversible forms of dementia are jets heading to the same airport. And there is never a smooth landing.

I am not going to spend time reviewing the nuances of the various conditions and suspected causes, because all the irreversible dementias are awful. I suggest checking out the Alzheimer's Association website if you want to get more information, in layman's terms, on a specific form of dementia.[5]

The core issue for family members is focusing on *what to expect* and *what to do* in response to the dementia, regardless of its title or how it goes about its systematic attack on the brain.

The Mayo Clinic says there are five stages typically associated with Alzheimer's disease. Others break it down into three, seven, or some other grouping. But the Mayo version makes sense to me, so I'm going with their take on it.[6]

The first is the *preclinical* phase. This can go on for years without any symptoms apparent to the person with the disease, and the signs are equally hidden to the person's family and close friends. But the damage is being done, like a slow leak in the roof dripping down the interior walls and slowly undermining the foundation. Deposits of a protein called amyloid beta are getting stored in the brain, causing inevitable damage. There isn't something simple like a blood test to diagnose Alzheimer's disease. A doctor makes the diagnosis largely based on some cognitive tests and what he observes in interacting with the patient. (Alzheimer's disease can only be conclusively confirmed by an autopsy. But what's the point of that, unless a body is being donated for scientific research?)

Alzheimer's typically starts when a person is in their mid to late sixties. Not always, but that is a general rule. People who show symptoms before they hit age sixty-five are considered to have early-onset Alzheimer's. The 5 percent of Alzheimer's sufferers who have the early onset form of the malady can develop symptoms as early as their forties or fifties. It is just flat-out tragic to get the disease that early in life.

After the preclinical phase comes *mild cognitive impairment* or MCI. The National Institute on Aging summarizes MCI as

a condition in which people have more memory or other thinking problems than normal for their age, but their symptoms do not interfere with their everyday lives. Older people with MCI are at greater risk for developing Alzheimer's, but not all of them do. Some may even go back to normal cognition. Studies are underway to learn why some people with MCI progress to Alzheimer's and others do not. The problems associated with MCI may also be caused by certain medications, cerebrovascular disease (which affects blood vessels that supply the brain), and other factors. *Some of the problems brought on by these conditions can be managed or reversed.* (Emphasis added, because I think that last sentence is a very big deal!)[7]

MCI is marked by becoming a bit more forgetful, getting a bit befuddled about things that used to be easy. MCI can include walking to the car and forgetting where you were intending to go. It can include lapses in judgment, falling for telemarketing scams, and making odd purchases and bad decisions. People who know you will suspect something is a wee bit wrong if you are suffering from MCI.

When I was working for a congressman, a man came into my office to complain about the post office. He was livid that the post office had refused to sell him a money order—after he mentioned to the clerk that he had won the German lottery but had to "pay the taxes in advance" before a large number of deutsche marks would be wired back to him.

"Sir, this is called a scam. The postal service is doing you a favor by not selling you the money order," I said.

"I won it fair and square, and I want my winnings!" he snapped.

"Sir, do you recall ever entering a German lottery?"

Pause.

"No, but I still won. They told me!"

"They are trying to steal from you."

"Are you going to help me or not?"

"Please trust me on this, I *am* helping you."

He had a few zesty and surprisingly creative profanities to lob my direction before he stormed off. I suspect mild cognitive impairment.

(We will revisit MCI and possible future treatments in the zany and somewhat scandalous chapter titled "Are You Smoking Something?")

But the good news is that a diagnosis of MCI doesn't necessarily lead to a diagnosis of Alzheimer's disease. Head to a doctor if you notice that a loved one has even mild signs of trouble with memory or thinking. Early intervention may help. The bad news is that if Alzheimer's is at work, then you are stuck with the harsh reality that it's a disease that can't be reversed.

The next step in the Alzheimer's progression is *mild dementia*. This is often the point when either the person with the disease or a concerned friend or family member realizes that something weird is definitely going on.

When Karin wished us a very merry Christmas during Easter dinner, we knew something was up. And that suspicion was compounded when she was playing Scrabble with Dale one day and placed a word on the board that wasn't connected to any other word. Karin had been playing this game for decades, and if she had been well, she would have known this was not how the game is played.

"Mom, are you sure you want to play that word there?" Dale asked.

"It gives me the most points," Karin replied.

Which was true, but a bit unorthodox according to the standard conventions of the game. It would be the equivalent of continuing to send your baseball team out to bat when all three prior batters had struck out.

In many ways, we found the mild dementia phase to be the hardest phase (but by no means the most heartbreaking). It was so hard because Karin would alternate between admitting that she was having some trouble with her memory and basic tasks, and then reacting strongly to any hint that she was anything other than a strong and independent woman.

When Dale suggested that perhaps her mom would enjoy having lunch at the local senior center that was mere steps from her apartment, Karin replied crisply, "I still know how to cook. Besides, all of the people who go there are old."

"But Mom, you're eighty-four."

"*I am?* Are you *sure?*"

Below are the kinds of things to look out for in the mild stage of Alzheimer's—

Forgetting recent events: "Mom, did you enjoy watching the Rose Parade yesterday?"

"Was it on? I missed it!"

(She had watched it with us.)

Asking the identical question again and again: "How old are you now?"

(She asked that every few minutes during our son's birthday party.)

Getting overwhelmed by normal tasks, such as trying to pay the bills or balance the checkbook.

(Karin would ask us to drive her to the bank so the tellers could do it for her.)

Getting lost while driving in familiar areas: "Dale, I'm calling from that little red phone you gave me. I was going to the grocery store, but I can't find it. I don't know what happened. I don't know where I am. Can you come and get me?"

(This happened with increasing frequency. She would drive for hours, utterly incapable of remembering streets and places she had known for decades.)

Trouble with expressing what they are trying to communicate: "I need one of those things for the eggs. The cooking thing. The holding thing. Oh, I just can't think of it!"

Calling things by the wrong name: "I want some of those olives for my oatmeal."

(She meant to say *raisins*.)

When Karin was still living independently, but definitely in the mild stage of the disease, she would routinely call me when she couldn't recall how to operate the remote control for her television. She might call five times in the same evening.

"This is so frustrating, but I can't seem to get the TV to turn on."

"That's okay. I'll walk you through it. Are you holding the remote?"

"Yes."

"Okay, do you see the top button on the right-hand side? The one that says 'on?'"

"Mine says 'redial.'"

"Um, that's actually the . . . wrong remote. How about if I just drive over and help you out?"

"I hate to put you out. But that would be nice of you."

It wasn't that far of a drive. And it also gave us a chance to check in on her.

You might also be perplexed by the odd statements your loved one makes.

Karin told us, "Someone keeps breaking into my home and putting strange clothes in my closet."

That would be a highly peculiar form of burglary, carried out by a miscreant failing to grasp the point of his or her profession. It would be such an odd crime, the police would have to coin a new term for it: *Misdemeanor Robin Hood breaking and entering.* But it turned out that the clothes were all items that she had worn for years. We checked just to make sure she hadn't brought someone else's clothes from the laundry room.

The next step is *moderate dementia.*

This is usually the longest stage of the disease. This is the stage Karin has been in for the past few years. Once your loved one is sliding into the moderate stage, you're up against the hard fact that she simply cannot safely live on her own.

You know broccoli goes in the refrigerator, not the bedroom closet. And you don't open a can of soup and put it in the cupboard. But Karin started making those kinds of mistakes when she was living in her own apartment. Those actions spoke volumes. They were like the engine warning light coming on, or the smoke detector starting to chirp. It signaled a serious condition. I'll fill you in later as to what unfolded when we decided she could not live on her own anymore, but for now, let me just say that it launched us on a wild ride that continues to this day. There are a thousand things you have to deal with when you take over the management of someone else's life, and that is even more true when they don't remember where any of their important papers might be (or whether they have such papers to begin with) or when you find a mason jar holding thirty sets of keys.

The moderate stage can also bring increasingly odd behaviors. Dale kept finding tissues and napkins ripped in half and tucked away in drawers and other odd little corners of Karin's apartment. Shredding tissues or napkins is a common habit of people afflicted with dementia. Hiding things is also a common activity. When her cell phone disappeared, we spent an hour going through every nook and cranny until we discovered it in the bathroom, in a drawer in a small box hidden under tubes of toothpaste and medical ointments.

It was in the early part of the moderate stage that Karin forgot her address and phone number. She would forget which daughter she was talking to. She was surprised to learn that she had grandchildren and wondered why she had never met them before. She repeatedly remarked that she had never been to our house before, when she had been in our home many hundreds of times over the previous two decades. And it was during this stage when Dale and Karin had regular conversations about her neighbor, whom I have dubbed "the Senior Citizen Formerly Known as Esther."

By way of background, the Senior Citizen Formerly Known as Esther is not in the witness protection program, and her name has always been, and continues to be, Esther. But Karin was convinced otherwise.

"I'll need a ride to church and so will that lady who lives down the hall from me."

"Do you mean Esther?" Dale asked.

"Well, she calls herself that, but it isn't her name," Karin would reply.

"Why do you think she calls herself Esther if that isn't her name?"

"Because everyone keeps calling her that!" replied Karin, exasperated with the whole bunch of us.

As the moderate stage progressed, Karin also began to hallucinate. She was deeply concerned that random children kept appearing in her apartment. She would wander the halls of her senior apartment complex, knocking on doors to ask if any of her neighbors knew where the absentee parents might have gone. This caused quite a few raised eyebrows, especially when Karin posed the question rather late in the evening.

But put yourself in her position for a moment: Wouldn't *you* be alarmed if you suddenly found unattended kids in your house? A dozen questions would swirl through your mind. How did they get here? Why are they in my home? Am I supposed to be babysitting them? What should I feed them? How long will they be here? What happened to their parents? Should I phone the police? What are their names? Who let them in? Shouldn't they be in school? Why are they so quiet? Are they supposed to be at the home of the lady who keeps calling herself Esther, even though that isn't her name?

Karin called us about the children, and we drove over to see what was going on.

Sitting on her sofa were six stuffed animals, all arranged to look at the television.

Her doctor prescribed a mix of medications to deal with the hallucinations. As a nice side effect, they also made her sleepy at night so she could get back into a more normal sleep cycle.

It is in the moderate stage of Alzheimer's that you might also notice your loved one dressing in wildly mismatched garments, mistaking pajamas for a blouse or a bathrobe for a coat. They may put on multiple pairs of socks. They may waltz into the living room attired for a day at a nudist beach.

Get used to being surprised. A lot.

For many people afflicted with Alzheimer's, the confusion gets worse toward sunset. This is called *sundowning*. No one really knows why it happens, but it is a commonly observed phenomenon. Maybe they are just worn-out at the end of the day. Maybe the change in light triggers something. People put forth all kinds of theories. Bottom line, be aware of it and brace for increased confusion, agitation, irritation, or disorientation at that time of day.

Your sundowning loved one might start cursing like a sailor. (It might become a bit disruptive at the church potluck.) Just bear in mind they can't help it.

One evening, a typically gentle and kind resident at Festive Acres took a look around the living room and told her five housemates, "I don't know who *any* of you people are, so get the *(exceptionally bad word)* out of my house!"

This immediately gave the staff the opportunity to employ their skills in the fine art of redirection.

Some people begin to pace. Or raise their voice. Or believe someone has stolen something from them. Or tell the imaginary children that they really must leave. When that happens, it's time to steer your loved one to bed or adjust the temperature or close the blinds and turn on the lights (that helps some people) or put on some soothing music or reassure them (you can speak calming words, hold their hand, read them a short story, or even sing a favorite song or hymn). And check with the doctor to see if a medication might help. You might also want to make sure that they are not napping for hours at a time in the afternoon. If they are too rested, falling asleep at night can be even harder for them. This is a big list, but by no means is it exhaustive. It is a matter of trying lots of stuff and seeing what works.

And if that isn't hard enough, you need to be prepared for a personality change in your loved one. Mom might start crying a lot for no clear reason. You do your best to rule things out—is she tired, or too hot or too cold? Does she need to sleep? Use the restroom? Did she have an accident before she could get to the restroom? Is she hungry? Sometimes there is something you can address, and sometimes it is just one more difficult twist in the progression of the disease. Again, try various things and see what might work. It may be that nothing really works, and so you adjust to the new dynamic.

Some families have to deal with hitting and biting. A study of German nursing homes revealed that about one third of caregivers feels severely stressed by violence and aggression.[8] Why do patients act out like this?

Well, let's suppose you got kidnapped. Wouldn't you fight back? Wouldn't you make a run for it if you saw an opening? Well, what if Mom or Dad is confused by the new surroundings and is in a panic? Nothing makes sense to them, and so they act out.

I befriended a guy named Phil. He had to go to a rehabilitation hospital to recover from an injury. I knew he didn't have family nearby, so I went to visit him.

His face lit up when he saw me. Then he looked around the room and motioned me over so he could whisper.

"Get me out of here. They're trying to kill me!"

"Phil, the doctor wants you here for a bit so you can get better," I replied.

"My keys are in the drawer. Just pull my van around to the front. I'll give you five minutes and then make a run for it."

"Phil, I can't take you out of here."

"Of course you can! That little nurse weighs 120 pounds. You can take her out."

"Phil, I can't do that. But is there anything I can do to make you more comfortable?"

He paused for a moment.

"A cheeseburger. The food here is horrible. That's how they get rid of us. The terrible food."

So I went down the hall and asked the nurse if I could bring Phil a burger.

"We don't allow outside food for the patients, so I can't give you a green light," she replied. But then she added, "If you do go get something and bring it back, I'm going to assume you're the one eating it while you visit your friend." And she gave me a wink and a smile.

Phil really did believe that someone had set him up for the hospitalization and that it was part of a dark conspiracy to kill him. That kind of paranoia is certainly one possible scenario for acting out, but who knows what is triggering the behavior?

Are they in pain? Scared? Tired? If they have a pattern of volatile behavior in response to a specific stimulus, then deal with the trigger. Is Dad livid when he is awakened for breakfast? Then by all means, let him sleep in and eat later. Does an evening shower or bath set him off? Try earlier in the day.

If someone attacks the television when a tense scene comes on, switch the channel to old *Lawrence Welk* reruns, or *I Love Lucy*, or something calming and beautiful like *Aerial America*.

Do they act out when it is noisy? Or when you switch from a normal routine? Be a bit of a Sherlock Holmes and look for clues. Many family members and caregivers report that they can calm a patient down by discovering and addressing an underlying issue.

It isn't unusual to get pushback when it's time for a bath or shower.

"I just had a bath and I am *not* taking another one!"

Wouldn't you throw a hissy fit if you just had a bath five minutes ago and your smarty-pants daughter said it was time for another one? Of course, it *wasn't* five minutes ago. It was two days ago. But Mom or Dad's reality is quite different from yours. They might think you're acting like a complete dingbat for trying to make them take multiple baths in rapid succession.

Your loved one can also lose all sense of time.

"Well, Mom, we should get you ready for bed."

"*Bed?* It's morning! I just got up! I think I'll cook some eggs."

If nothing else works, you may need to consult with a doctor about medication. There are downsides and health risks associated with some of these medications, but dealing with Alzheimer's means considering trade-offs.

The last phase of Alzheimer's disease is the *severe phase*. Generally speaking, this time is marked by the loss of ability to have anything that would pass for real communication. Your loved one may say some random words or even repeat a rote phrase, but their communication is pretty much incomprehensible. People in this stage can no longer take care of personal hygiene or use the toilet without assistance. They will require help getting dressed. They will likely lose the ability to feed themselves. Their mobility will decline, and they may no longer be able to walk without assistance—or walk at all. As time rolls on they can become completely bedridden. They will no longer be able to control bodily functions. Tragically, they can lose the ability to swallow food.

People can move through these stages at different speeds, and many do not make it into the severe stage before they pass away.

Several of Karin's former housemates in her assisted-living home were in the moderate stage when their heart simply gave out, a stroke took them, or they never recovered from a brief bout with pneumonia. These were people who, right up to their last week or so, had been able to engage in at least some chats that sort of made sense, could use coloring books, or put a puzzle together (as long as you helped them a lot, the pieces were really big, and there weren't very many of them). These were lovely people who would break into a smile when they got a visitor, hold hands with a friend, and enjoy having a slice of birthday cake.

Yes, they were confused a lot. But they were happy most of the time. Little things and little routines clearly brought them joy. While this terrible disease had robbed them of much of their memory and diminished their ability to function on their own, it did not have the chance to hit them with the full force of the condition. One day I asked the administrator of Karin's assisted-living facility roughly what percentage of his residents got so severely disabled by the disease that they had to be moved into a skilled-nursing facility.

"Almost none," he told me.

"But I thought you weren't equipped for the severe stage," I replied.

"They mostly just pass away here before they get to that stage," he said.

Honestly, that gives us a sense of peace. The most bitter and distressing phase of Alzheimer's is not the inevitable end, or even the most common end. It is true that skilled-nursing facilities have a large number of their beds filled with people in the last stage of a dementia disorder—rigid muscles, unable to speak, wasting slowly away in a world that has shrunk to the size of a mattress.

And the experience of one administrator in one assisted-living home is more anecdote than data. But still, it is also what I have seen with my own eyes. Karin's housemates were doing relatively well in the moderate stage, then had a brief illness, or simply went to bed and woke up in the presence of God.

We don't know the path the disease will take with Karin. Alzheimer's disease progresses at widely different rates. Typically, people live about eight to ten years after getting diagnosed. But some people have been known to live more than two decades after diagnosis. So we simply don't know. We *do* know that someday her mind and body will be restored beyond her wildest dreams, because there is a good God and he has a great life waiting for his children after this life ends.

> Jesus said to her, "I am the resurrection and the life; he who believes in Me will live even if he dies, and everyone who lives and believes in Me will never die. Do you believe this?" She said to Him, "Yes, Lord; I have believed that You are the Christ, the Son of God, even He who comes into the world."
>
> John 11: 25–27 (NASB)

# SIX

# Money Matters

K arin had always been generous to mission organizations, various ministries, and even political organizations. But she began rashly giving away money to just about any organization that called her. And boy, did they call when she was still living on her own.

"Hello, Mrs. Hastings. We are calling on behalf of Babies Born with No Teeth, and we would like to supply them with dentures. Can we count on you for twenty-five dollars?"

"Well, that sounds very nice. Let me get my credit card," she would inevitably reply.

So Dale and I found ourselves lugging Karin's copious amounts of mail to our place so we could plod through the paper blizzard. Many of the organizations were clearly scams, even if they managed to somehow scrape by the most basic laws governing this kind of stuff. It was almost like they were designed to prey on confused senior citizens. I have to believe there is a special room in hell for the people who create these kinds of organizations, and it would be poetic justice if the flames were fueled by a billion tons of junk mail.

PAST DUE NOTICE, my eye!

We tried the trick of writing "MOVED, NO FORWARD-ING ADDRESS" and dropping the stacks of mail back into the mailbox. But the pleas for money still came, much like those recurring swarms of locusts that inevitably return to ravage Africa, only more annoying and with bulk mail privileges. I resorted to writing "DECEASED" on the mail, even though it technically violated numerous biblical directives about honesty. But the junk mail still flowed like a mighty Amazon River of paper.

Once those junk mail people get a dime from you, or just get a whiff of a possibility that you may even remotely consider sending some loot, they latch on with the tenacity of a starving rodent that has pounced on the planet's last Cheeto. It would take a crowbar to pry them off a befuddled senior citizen, or perhaps even a few cruise missiles. (Note: the Pentagon will turn you down, even though they do sound pretty sympathetic on the phone.)

So, lacking advanced firepower or any other viable options, I just had her mail forwarded to our house and bought a commercial-sized shredder. I suspect our mail carrier secretly hates me, because I must have doubled his workload. I hope he never bothers to glance at the senders of the voluminous correspondence, because I don't want to face him after he realizes he routinely delivers mail from the Society for the Preservation of the Prancing Newt or "urgent alerts" from the American Association of Extremely Retired Persons Who Will Blow a Major Gasket If Congress Even *Thinks* About Touching Social Security.

On the plus side, in the event the earth is plunged into another ice age I will have enough free fuel for a bonfire that never goes out.

It is vital to get at least shared control of your loved one's finances before they are no longer able to make an informed and legally acceptable decision. There is a massive benefit to Mom or Dad willingly bringing you on board while they still have the mental capacity to add you to their accounts. It is an utterly different thing if they don't grant that permission and then get so far along the dementia pathway that you need to gain conservatorship (think "hideous legal nightmare that could cost you the equivalent of the gross domestic product of Honduras by the time you are finished").

It is actually a pretty straightforward process to have Mom or Dad sign a power of attorney form allowing you to make financial decisions on their behalf. And it is quite easy to go down to the bank and get your name added to the checking account. But the process is probably going to be the least of your problems.

"I am doing *fine* on my own, and I certainly don't need my daughter to write checks for me! You might recall that I changed your diapers just fine without your help. Besides, if anything happened to me, your dad could take over."

Um, wrong. Karin's spouse was already well down the road into moderate Alzheimer's disease, which is why, at eighty-six years old, he got out of bed at 2:00 a.m. and wandered outside to find a big rig truck he could drive to Oregon to pick up a load of wood. But Karin simply could not accept the diagnosis and fashioned a hundred different, wildly implausible explanations for his condition.

Her excuse for this incident? "He was just tired."

It can be exceptionally difficult for your parent to admit they need your help. And the excuses, rationalizations, and non sequiturs can roll forth like waves crashing on the beach.

"I've been balancing my checkbook longer than you've been alive."

(When we peeked at the check register, it was a random distribution of numbers with nothing that resembled a running total.)

"Yes, I've been a bit forgetful lately, but that doesn't mean I need you to meddle in my affairs."

(Code for *I fear losing my independence*.)

"If I think I need help, I'll tell you."

(Code language for *never*.)

"You sure are getting bossy these days."

(Code language for *I am still the parent, and you're getting too big for your britches!*)

"Boy, the Visa people have started charging me a lot of late fees these days. I've never been late with a bill in my life! I'm going to give those people a piece of my mind."

(You might find a lot of righteous indignation at things that are clearly her fault, including the shut-off warning from the power company and the fact that the car's gas tank has mysteriously emptied itself.)

"Help me find the checkbook. Someone must have moved it again."

Dale handled the situation very deftly.

"Mom, I'm not saying you can't pay your own bills or shop for what you need. But suppose something happened? What if you got the flu, and Dad was sick, and someone needed to be able to take care of things until you got better? I should be able to write checks for you if you're not able to take care of things."

"Well, I guess that makes sense," Karin replied.

We printed off a general durable power of attorney form I found online that was approved for use in our state. The durable form is the best bet, since it is not limited by time.

An explanation is in order here. Signing a power of attorney (POA) form does not mean you need an attorney or that you are an attorney or that the person gaining power is an attorney or that an attorney has to get within a five-block radius of your loved one or that this is going to cost you a boatload of money because the word *attorney* is mentioned.

Indeed, ours cost us nothing more than the twenty bucks a notary public charged us to witness the signatures.

A POA is a document with a bunch of pretty standard language that, boiled down, means Person A is allowing Person B to make certain choices when Person A cannot make those choices for himself. The person who is deemed the attorney-in-fact can have all the legal training of a zucchini and still use the POA on behalf of Person A.

The POA form I chose had a host of options Karin could either approve or disallow: real estate transactions, stocks and bonds, tangible personal property, banking, insurance, claims and litigation, government benefits such as social security and Medicare, and even commodity transactions. (Karin did not deal in soybean futures, but if she did, we would have been prepared.) Indeed, the list covered about everything except health care issues and running for mayor. (Different forms are required for both of those.) The last box on the form was an "all of the above" option.

So, depending on which POA boxes get checked off, Mom or Dad can assign only some or pretty much all decision-making authority to you (or whichever trusted person is designated). It is a powerful document.

Karin checked the all-inclusive box that said Dale was empowered to do just about everything imaginable on Karin's behalf (short of declaring war on Cuba). And, importantly, she did so before the sad day her doctor had to certify that she was no longer legally competent to make any decisions beyond what kind of yogurt she wanted, or whether she was up to going for a walk.

(You can sign a POA long before you need anyone to act on your behalf, and it's actually a very good idea to do so. Spouses can do this for each other. So grab a couple extra forms for yourselves.)

Signing the POA doesn't mean you must hand over your life to someone else as soon as the ink is dry. It means you are empowering a trusted person to act in your stead with your best interests in mind when you aren't able to act.

A classic example is when you are hospitalized and someone needs to keep paying the bills. It is more like sharing power than giving up power. Because what if you slipped into a coma? Or, in Karin's case, slipped into dementia?

The durable (ongoing, as opposed to terminating on a certain date) POA gives Dale the power, and also the legal responsibility, to act in her mom's best interests for as long as Karin is alive. Yes, Dale has access to her mom's money. No, Dale can't use it to take a trip to France. It is her legal responsibility to do the right thing for Karin. There are serious criminal penalties for elder abuse, and financial crimes committed upon a person with dementia are certainly abuse.

Legally, Dale can spend money, deposit checks, cash checks, sell real estate, tap an IRA, enter into a contract, file insurance claims, and all that kind of stuff on her mom's behalf. And she has had to do all of that in the past few years.

Dale's obligation means not mingling her mom's funds with ours (Karin has a separate checking account, which has her and Dale's names on it). We keep a record of how we spend the money, and the check register is available to either family members or agents of the state. The United Nations could have a look at it for all we care. Indeed, we keep better records than they do.

It is important to note that a POA is not a will. The POA dies with the person who authorized it, and then the will kicks in. If Mom or Dad hasn't created a will, that is an entirely different animal. You can't fix that with a simple POA. If someone passes away without creating a will, then everything defaults to state law for the distribution of the estate. I really don't want to get further into details about wills, because it doesn't take long for legal stuff to make me curl up into a fetal position and start whimpering.

Ideally, a highly trusted family member, or some other dependable and willing person, is designated as the POA. (Also sometimes referred to as the *agent*, but nothing covert is involved. No one gives you a pen that turns into a flame-thrower or anything cool like that.)

But because Mom or Dad is free to name *anyone* as the agent of their POA, they might. And that includes someone shady who worms his or her way into their confidence and intends to rip them off. You need to know what is going on, and whether Mom or Dad has handed a boatload of authority to someone who can harm them.

I knew an elderly lady who was "befriended" by a business associate who managed to use the POA to make all kinds of horrendous financial decisions for the person he was "helping." Lots of money disappeared, and the lady's business was taken over by this unscrupulous guy. The family found out about it too late, and Mr. Scam Artist had vanished.

If you feel that someone is ripping off your loved one, there are elder abuse laws on the books, and the local district attorney has staff who should know what to do. Contact law enforcement or the social service office. They can either take action or get you in touch with the people who can. But you really don't want to deal with this after the damage has already been done.

Sadly, a great deal of elder abuse is perpetrated by a family member. This is one of the many reasons there is a place called hell, and I think there are some hotter rooms reserved for people who prey upon confused and vulnerable senior citizens.

A POA can be revoked by the person who created it, as long as they are still competent. If Mom or Dad hasn't created a POA, and they aren't mentally competent to do so now, you may need to go through a legal process to become their conservator or guardian. Sorry to be the bearer of bad news, but it is probably going to cost at least a few thousand dollars—more if someone contests it.

Properly used, a POA is a wonderful tool that empowers you to help Mom or Dad. It is inexpensive, fast to create, and easy to implement. Make a POA one of your top priorities. Your next priority is to get similar authority for health care issues, and that is what we cover next.

# SEVEN

# I'm Feeling Fine

Similar to the general/financial POA is a medical power of attorney, which is also known as a health care proxy or a POA for health care. There may be a somewhat different title depending on what state you live in, but the basic idea is the same. Person A (Mom) can designate Person B (you) to make health care decisions if Person A is unable to do so. As with the financial POA, this document can only be completed while Mom or Dad is still mentally competent to sign it.

Closely tied to this document is the advance health care directive. This document allows someone to spell out their wishes, such as "don't you *dare* hook me up to all those tubes when it's my time to go!" But the language typically has more technical medical jargon.

Your doctor will have this form available. The hospital will have this form available. Every medical facility within a ten-county area will have a stack of these forms. You can also find them online at a site like Everplans.[1] Advance health care directives are routinely made available at health fairs and events targeted at senior citizens so that these critically important documents can be taken home and shoved in a drawer and forgotten, or turned into scratch paper, or otherwise studiously ignored by huge numbers of senior citizens who are uncomfortable thinking about worst-case scenarios.

One doctor told me he often hears patients say, "I'm not going to fill out one of those things, because I know someone who signed one and then keeled over dead." I am not making this up.

There is no such thing as being jinxed by signing an advance directive. But people can get weirdly superstitious about this. So you need to have this conversation with Mom and Dad while they can still make an informed decision.

One doctor told me he wished that filling out an advance health care directive was mandatory for everyone enrolling in Medicare. (*That* would certainly increase compliance!)

"I don't care what decision my patients make, as long as they make their wishes known," he said. "If they want every treatment under the sun to prolong their life no matter what, fine. Just let me know. If they don't want extraordinary measures taken in certain circumstances, great. Just let me know. Let family know. Spell it out so we can respect your wishes. But the worst thing is when no one knows what you want, and family members are arguing in the hospital hallway outside your room."

The doctor went on to explain that he was emphatically *not* talking about physician-assisted suicide, or anything remotely close to it. It is about your making sure your wishes are known, and, therefore, carried out if you are incapacitated and can't communicate. A hospital administrator told me that, in the absence of knowing what you want, the medical profession is likely to take extraordinary and even outlandish measures not only to keep you alive but also to keep the attorneys at bay.

A doctor told me that most of his patients don't want to live on a respirator, unconscious, hooked up to a bunch of wires and monitors and intravenous fluids while they slowly and obliviously decline, with no real prospect of getting better. At that point, they would just like to let nature take its course. They want to be as pain-free as possible, they want hospice care, they don't want to feel like they can't breathe, and they don't want to be gripped by panic.

"We can offer excellent end-of-life care," he said. "We can manage the pain. But if they don't document their wishes, they are placing a huge burden on their loved ones. The family can be wracked by guilt, or too emotionally paralyzed to make a decision. A lot of really unsound and actually cruel medical 'care' is driven by the fear of being sued. I want my patients to be in charge of these decisions, and that means filling out a directive. And it isn't chiseled in stone. You can alter it at any time. The key is simply this—tell us what you want."

Dale's parents didn't have that conversation with her.

This isn't unusual. It is more of a general rule. The journal *Health Affairs* reported that in 150 studies conducted on nearly 800,000 people between 2011 and 2016, researchers learned that just 36 percent had completed advance directives or a living will.[2]

I am part of the problem. I have been offered the advance directive form dozens of times—I have even taken the paperwork home a few times—but somehow I have just not gotten around to it. I have had conversations with my wife, but I haven't put my wishes down on paper. And I am a writer by profession.

I tell myself I will get around to it, especially if I am diagnosed with a serious condition. But, alarmingly, the Agency for Healthcare Research and Quality reported several years ago that the *majority* of "severely or terminally ill patients" had not quite managed to get around to completing advance directives.[3] What in the world are they thinking?

"Yeah, I may have an inoperable tumor, and the doctor has given me only three months to live, but there are some *Seinfeld* episodes I wanted to see again. So I've been busy. Planning to get around to it, though. Probably after the episode where Jerry gets the first-class ticket and Elaine gets stuck in coach."

One day, Dale was helping clean out her mom's closet when she stumbled across a large blue binder with a cover sheet that read, "The Eugene and Karin Hastings Family Trust." It had been created in 1998.

Dale had had no idea it existed. By the time she found it, her mother was well down the Alzheimer's path and probably couldn't have had a lucid conversation about it. Dale started leafing through it and was surprised to discover that she had been named a trustee. And in poring through the numerous sections and pages, Dale was particularly astonished to find that her parents had deemed *her* their health care proxy if they were not able to serve that function for one another. The document elaborately detailed what medical interventions they did or did not wish for based upon specified health benchmarks.

Um, it might have been a good idea to mention it to Dale.

But at least we stumbled upon it right when we needed it (thank you, God) because Dale's father, already suffering from a pretty bad stage of Alzheimer's, got a stubborn infection and had to be hospitalized that very week.

It seemed like we were practically living at the hospital for weeks. One day, when Dale and I were kind of punchy from lack of sleep and involved in a discussion with a doctor, we didn't notice that Karin had stepped out of the room. She had heard the phone ringing in the nurse's station and saw that all the nurses were occupied with patients. So Karin, who had once been a charge nurse, took control of the situation by answering the phone. She was in the process of scheduling an admission when one of the nurses ran up to the desk and snatched the phone away.

"You can't answer our phones!" she sputtered.

"Well, *you* weren't at your station!" Karin retorted.

We heard the commotion and retrieved Karin before she could write up the nurse for an infraction.

Dale's dad was put on intravenous antibiotics and began to respond. He could take short walks around the hallways. He demanded to go home. But the doctors couldn't get the condition fully under control. The moment he went off the antibiotics, the infection roared back. Over the course of a few weeks he spiraled downward and finally slipped into a condition where he couldn't communicate, had no possibility of improving, but could be artificially kept alive. He would need a feeding tube and other extreme measures.

We consulted his advance directive.

"I, Eugene Edward Hastings . . . hereby grant to my agent full power and authority to make health care decisions for me to the same extent that I could make such decisions for myself if I had the capacity to do so. In exercising this authority, my agent shall make health care decisions that are consistent with my desires as stated in this document or otherwise made known to my agent, including, but not limited to, my desires concerning obtaining or refusing or withdrawing life-prolonging care, treatment, services, and procedures.

"I desire that mere biological existence not be the sole criteria in making decisions concerning my health care. I desire that the nature of that existence be taken into account as well . . . the focal point of the decision should be the prognosis as to the reasonable possibility of return to cognitive and sapient life, as distinguished from the forced continuation of biological vegetative existence. I desire that my life be prolonged only when it does not mean a mere suspension of the act of dying but contemplates, at the very least, a remission of symptoms enabling a return toward a normal, functioning, integrated existence."

It went on like that for several pages, offering highly specific guidance for numerous scenarios. It was technical and lawyerly and wordy and often redundant, but it took on the beauty of Shakespeare's sonnets. It was a gift. It didn't require my wife to make a wrenching decision and live with a constant, nagging doubt about whether or not she did the right thing. It simply required us to hand a copy to the nurse and say, "These are his wishes. Please make sure that the doctor and all the treating medical staff know."

Gene was in the rehabilitation hospital for about five weeks, slowly slipping away day by day. Dale's mom, confident in her professional abilities, wanted to take him home and nurse him back to health. At her stage of dementia, she couldn't understand the reality of the situation.

The doctor was very gentle.

"Karin, that will not be successful. Let us do what we can for him."

But the doctor knew where this was headed. And he also knew that the medical POA listed Karin as primary only as long as she was capable of serving in that role. If she was not, Dale was empowered to take on the role of "agent."

One late evening, with family members gathered around his bed, Dale's dad took his last breath and was received into the presence of God. It was a difficult time, but it was made much less wrenching because there really was no "decision" for us to make. Gene had already decided and had spelled out his wishes in very specific terms. (Thank you, Gene, for having the foresight to do this.)

You need to know: Does Dad wish to be resuscitated if he stops breathing? Or only under certain conditions? Does Mom want to be put on a respirator? Should other artificial life support be employed? How about a feeding tube? Under what circumstances? What if two doctors concur that Mom or Dad is not going to emerge from unconsciousness, even though the body can be kept alive? What if siblings do not agree?

These are hard discussions to have, but vital.

If the window has closed to create an advance directive, then family should discuss these issues before a crisis hits. You don't want to be forced into snap decisions in the heat of the moment. Do what you think your loved one would want, and do what you think is honestly in their best interest. We are all mortal. No one gets out of here alive. You aren't taking the life of your parent. You are trying to do the best you can for them under the constraint of human mortality.

And bless you for being willing to step up.

EIGHT

# Laughter Is Good
for the Soul, Spleen,
and Mental Health

We stopped in at Festive Acres a bit before noon, and Karin greeted us with some big news.

"I just hitchhiked here, and they had lunch ready for me when I walked in!"

She had the kind of smile you would have if Buckingham Palace called to say they discovered you were the rightful heir to the throne, and you could legally banish Prince Charles if you felt like it.

"Well, that worked out great!" Dale replied.

Karin gave us a delighted grin.

We finished our visit, got into the car, and laughed. And then felt kind of bad about laughing. And then talked, once again, about the sensitive topic of laughing at anything connected to this cruel disease.

This brings me to why I decided to write this book. Believe me, I struggled mightily with the very idea of penning this manuscript, because my specific intent is to bring a dose of humor to a subject that is fraught with grief, pain, frustration, and loss. I began, and then abandoned, the idea no less than a dozen times. I returned to it because the reader reaction to a few short magazine articles convinced me that caregivers need to hear the stories of others in the same boat and *desperately* need to laugh about some of our shared experiences.

At the height of World War II, British Prime Minister Winston Churchill regularly set aside time to watch slapstick Groucho Marx films. He knew he couldn't take the nonstop stress of war. He knew he needed to laugh. I believe he was wise.

If you are caring for someone who has Alzheimer's or another form of dementia, you are in a pressure cooker. Even if you aren't the daily caregiver, you love someone whose mind is being slowly whittled away by this disease process. You bear a great weight.

Dale and I never laugh *at* Karin or anyone with Alzheimer's. We laugh at the utterly unexpected comments. We smile at the absurdities that take us completely off guard. We laugh so we won't cry, or sometimes we laugh and cry at the same time.

Karin: "I'm left-handed, but I like to bat with my right."

Those kinds of out-of-the-blue comments can necessitate that I excuse myself and leave the room for a few minutes so I don't just crack up in front of her.

You will have many times of mourning, of grieving the inexorable loss of your loved one. When it is clear that one more precious memory has faded into the gray fog, you swallow hard and perhaps tear up. That event Mom could still talk about last month now draws a blank stare. It is a stabbing reminder that your shared memory is no longer shared. That hurts. And it is normal and healthy to grieve that loss. But you can't just experience a relentless sense of loss, or you will have no reservoir of strength for the journey still to come.

Don't feel guilty when Mom or Dad says something that is so surprising or absurd that your impulse is to giggle. Embrace it. Consider the spontaneous laughter a blessing from the God who designed you with the capacity to laugh. You are not being mean or disrespectful. You are not being a jerk. You are relieving stress, and it is healthy.

Winston Churchill knew he would be crushed under the weight of the war if he did not take time to laugh. There is nothing funny about the bloodshed and awful destruction of war. The prime minister was not laughing *at* the hostilities or the suffering of his nation. It was not inappropriate for him to seek mental relief or to find some levity in the midst of all that was so terribly sad.

So cut yourself some slack. Not only is it good for you to laugh, it is good for your loved one. If it is still possible to joke with Mom or Dad, by all means do so. I have a running joke with Karin regarding my looks. If Karin says to my wife, "Your hair looks nice today," I will run my fingers through my balding head and ask, "Do I get any praise for my hair?"

"Which one of them?" she quips, grinning like an imp.

There will likely come a time when we can no longer banter with her. So we are going to enjoy it while we can. We have friends who have already walked this journey, and they have advised us to celebrate everything you still *can* do together instead of focusing so intensely on what Mom or Dad *can't* do anymore.

But what if your loved one is now so advanced in the disease that she doesn't recognize you, cannot speak, and can't even leave her bed? What do you do when no interaction is possible? You hold her hand. Sing an old and familiar tune. Make sure that the staff is attentive to all of her physical needs.

And you go do things that bring you peace and joy. You keep living your life. Have coffee with a friend. Watch little kids play. Walk the dog. Read a funny book. Pray for strength. And fantasize about where you would banish Prince Charles if the palace ever calls with big news.

# NINE

# Notable Techniques for Beating a Dead Horse

If you should ever need to get a dead horse moving again, you can employ a variety of techniques. The most straightforward is to yell "giddy-up" in a commanding voice reminiscent of John Wayne. If the horse doesn't commence trotting (which is quite likely, since it's dead), you can try jabbing it with spurs. If those subtler methods don't produce the desired result, just grab any handy object and start pounding away on the immobile body of the lifeless mammal. Keep repeating these procedures for weeks, or even years, until the horse begins to stir.

Once you have succeeded in rousing the expired equine, you're ready to move on to the somewhat more difficult task of getting someone with Alzheimer's to recall the events you wish them to remember. (If I sound a bit testy, it's because I just witnessed someone doing this.)

Technique number one: get exasperated with them and say, "I just *told* you five minutes ago!" That will undoubtedly make them feel happy, while also jogging their memory.

Technique number two: ask, "Do you remember when (fill in details of the event you wish them to recall)?" If the person with Alzheimer's can't recall the event, express shock or disappointment and keep adding details until she snaps out of it.

Technique number three: talk to a third party about Mom or Dad's condition while Mom or Dad is right there. Say something like, "She asks me where the bathroom is twenty times a day!" You can also add a comment like, "I think she's just being obstinate." That has the added bonus of being demeaning.

I continue to be amazed and appalled at people who refuse to accept that the disease has imposed very real limits on the person with a neurocognitive disorder. I don't know if they think they can simply wish it away, if they are in abject denial, if they are completely uninformed about the condition, or if they are just inherently clueless. Or a jerk.

So in case any of them are listening, I'm going to speak slower and louder (a technique you can employ to help non-English speakers better understand you).

Now, l-i-s-t-e-n u-p. Never ask a question that contains the phrase "do you remember?" Because it is likely they often will not. And it is also likely that you will create alarm, frustration, or sadness by posing the question.

Next, don't tell stories from decades past, or even from yesterday, and expect them to share the memory. Think before you speak. Instead of putting them in the uncomfortable position of trying to recall a specific event, ask questions about the here and now.

"Do you like this soup?"

"Isn't that a pretty rose?"

"How are you feeling today?"

"Would you like to go for a walk?"

Or, make a statement.

"Janice and I went to a wonderful new bakery yesterday."

"I read a really good novel last night."

"I think the state legislature has lost its collective marbles and needs to be sent to its room."

Or, talk about the future.

"Mom, we're planning a vacation to go see the Corn Palace. It is a huge tourist attraction in Mitchell, South Dakota. It features 'uniquely designed corn murals,' according to the brochure Harold ordered. We could be going to Hawaii for two weeks, but Harold insisted on seeing a massive monument to the agriculture industry of South Dakota. I'm never doing his laundry again."

None of those questions or statements create a burden to remember something.

This does not mean you can never talk about the past. But it can mean you wait until your loved one brings it up.

Karin will often tell stories from her youth. The times she picked cranberries in Oregon. The day phone service came to her rural area. The day she entered college to earn her degree in nursing. It is wonderful when she can speak of a memory. And we have found ways to spark memories without using the forbidden word *remember*.

Dale will tell a story that does not directly involve her mom, but that might lead to something Karin does recall.

"Mom, we kids sure used to have fun picking strawberries together."

"They used to grow on our property!" Karin exclaims.

"That's right. But I'm not quite sure where."

"Just down the hill," replies Karin.

Bingo. It is often still possible to share memories, but we have to get there in a roundabout manner.

Don't make the mistake of trying to "help her remember." You can't. It is like trying to "help" a blind person see by pointing out "It's right smack in front of you. Just look harder!"

You cannot make it better. And the next chapter discusses why you should not be doing amateur experimentation for a cure.

# TEN

# Dr. Finster's Miracle Dementia-B-Gone Elixir

At some point you are going to meet a well-intentioned buffoon who is going to suggest an awesome new cure for Alzheimer's disease. He read it on the interweb, so it *must* be true.

Or you are going to cross paths with a charlatan who is only too happy to prey on your desperation. So, let's pause for yet another review of this disease, courtesy of the United States Department of Health and Humans Services, the umbrella organization for the National Institute on Aging (the main federal agency supporting and conducting Alzheimer's disease research).

Alzheimer's disease is an irreversible, progressive brain disorder that slowly destroys memory and thinking skills and, eventually, the ability to carry out the simplest tasks. In most people with Alzheimer's, symptoms first appear in their mid-

60s. Alzheimer's disease is the most common cause of dementia among older adults.

The disease is named after Dr. Alois Alzheimer. In 1906, Dr. Alzheimer noticed changes in the brain tissue of a woman who had died of an unusual mental illness. Her symptoms included memory loss, language problems, and unpredictable behavior. After she died, he examined her brain and found many abnormal clumps (now called amyloid plaques) and tangled bundles of fibers (now called neurofibrillary, or tau, tangles). These plaques and tangles in the brain are still considered some of the main features of Alzheimer's disease.

Another feature is the loss of connections between nerve cells (neurons) in the brain. Neurons transmit messages between different parts of the brain, and from the brain to muscles and organs in the body. *Although treatment can help manage symptoms in some people, currently there is no cure for this devastating disease.* (Emphasis added.)[1]

But the core of the matter is the line I quoted first: "Alzheimer's disease is an *irreversible*, *progressive* brain disorder that slowly destroys memory and thinking skills . . ."

It is horrible, and it isn't going to be halted. Dad is going to lose the ability to add and subtract even simple numbers. Mom will become baffled by buttons. Gran will need to switch to slip-on shoes because the tiny space in her brain that stored shoe-tying skills has become inaccessible. Language is inexorably slipping away, as if a thief is returning again and again to steal books from the library shelf of the mind.

The disease goes from bad to truly awful. The connections between nerve cells are fraying, falling apart, disconnecting. Think of it like short circuits in the brain. Sometimes your loved one can have a relatively good day and surprise you by seeming more lucid, just like when the lamp with the short circuit flickers back on. He might shock you by discussing something you did together last night or twenty years ago. Enjoy it, but don't start counting on it. And don't think of it as progress. It isn't. The right neurons managed to fire again, which is great. But the wiring is damaged and always deteriorating.

Our friend Peggy watched her mom decline over two decades. As is often the case, the disease began with what seemed to be simple absentmindedness and ended when Peggy's mom was unable to communicate, unable to get out of bed, and utterly cut off from the world.

Even if your loved one can benefit from a medication—and you should definitely seek a doctor's opinion in that regard—the disease can't be cured as of the day I write this. Governments and universities and pharmaceutical companies around the world are trying. But a cure isn't in sight.

Please ignore the home remedies and "cures" bouncing around the internet. If something really worked, it would be headline news all over the world. Don't let desperation make you a target for a scam. No "miracle food" or "weird new supplement" or "three-week natural cure" arrests Alzheimer's disease.

Quacks have been around for as long as people have sought cures. Mrs. Winslow's Soothing Syrup for Teething Children definitely quieted cranky babies back in the 1850s, because the concoction contained a substantial dose of morphine.[2] A 1910 issue of the *New York Times* reported that a chemical analysis revealed virtually all such "soothing syrups" contained "morphine sulphate, chloroform, morphine hydrochloride, codeine, heroin, powdered opium, cannabis indica," and often, to make the baby extra docile, a mix of several aforementioned ingredients.

Arsenic enjoyed quite a run as a component of Victorian cosmetics as well as an eighteenth-century cure for malaria. This would have been quite a lot of bang for the buck—were it not for the side effects of multisystem organ failure and death. The end could come fast or slow, depending on how much arsenic-laced face cream the ladies decided to slather on or how bad the mosquitos were that season.

The silvery liquid we know as mercury was wildly popular for thousands of years as a curative ointment for skin disorders, a way to heal fractures, prolong life, and for the twin functions as an aphrodisiac *and* contraceptive. It was also used to halt the spread of sexually transmitted diseases (which it actually did, mostly by killing off the sexually indiscriminate guys who used the mercury cure).[3]

Regrettably, many of the most outrageous historic medical practices were employed by doctors who really were trying to help but, because the scientific method had not gained traction yet, were woefully ignorant. But a massive amount of the quackery was peddled by scam artists who were only too happy to take money from the gullible, the desperate, and the suffering.

Medicine has made astonishing leaps in the past century. So talk to the doctors and other professionals, and let quacks stay in the realm of ducks.

# ELEVEN

# This Is Going to Hurt

My dentist gets away with stuff that would get anyone else arrested for assault with a deadly weapon. Every time I need dental work done, he comes at me with an enormous stabbing implement the size of the harpoon Captain Ahab plunged into the great white whale.

"Stop him! He's a madman!" I yell to the dental hygienist while I clamp my hands over my mouth.

She always pretends she doesn't hear me, which underscores a disturbing trend of citizen noninvolvement when others are in clear distress.

"Can't you use a smaller needle?" I ask my dentist every single time.

"Can't you just close your eyes or act your age?" he replies every single time.

After the initial shot of anesthetic, he has the gall to stick a screaming drill into my tooth. I have repeatedly called the anonymous tip line to turn him in to law enforcement, but they keep telling me that, since there was no intent to harm me, the act of oral mayhem is not a crime. (Then they tell me to just close my eyes and act my age, and they hang up on me.)

But my dentist is not the only guy who gets away with performing cruel and unusual actions upon my person. Once a year I make an appointment with my doctor for a complete physical exam, and each time he asks me to drop my trousers and cough twice while he reconnoiters, in a most awkward and distressing manner, a part of my anatomy that I would infinitely prefer he simply left alone and presumed was fine just the way it was.

The cops don't care about this outrage, either. My doctor has an actual license to do this stuff to me. It's that "intent" loophole, again.

In fact, there are all kinds of actions that would be punishable by fine or imprisonment in one context, but, in another setting, those same acts are applauded and get awarded by the mayor. If I smashed one of your windows, climbed into your house, ran into your bedrooms, and hauled your family out to the front lawn in the middle of the night, I would be charged with at several major crimes. When firefighters do the same thing, they earn your lasting gratitude.

That brings me to a difficult and recurring question we all struggle with at one time or another. Is there any purpose to the suffering we endure? What is God intending when pain crashes into our life?

The questions pour out along with our tears.

Does he care? If so, why doesn't he fix it? How can he say he loves us and then just watch our ongoing suffering? Is there any meaning to all the awfulness? Or is this just a random part of life? Or is the pain just a consequence of living in a fallen world, with no specific purpose for it?

I have struggled with the issue of pain all my life. And I do not have a great deal of patience with glib answers, especially from people who often are not in the midst of an agonizing problem when they offer commentary on the meaning of it all.

I have friends—really good, all-around awesome people who love God and love others—who have suffered from cancer, lost a child, watched a mom wither away with Alzheimer's disease, wrestled with mental illness, lost a spouse far too soon, endured the madness of an alcoholic parent, and the horrible list goes on.

I don't believe God *caused* any of it. But he didn't stop it either.

And that hurts.

Pain can feed our worst fears about God. That he is uncaring. Aloof. Immune to what assails us. Or, even worse, sadistic.

The minute I hear someone tell anyone else that "God brought (fill in the circumstance) into your life to help you learn (fill in the spiritual attribute—patience, empathy, compassion, or whatever)," I feel like delivering a fistful of my own "help" to help those would-be advisors about the danger of simplistic platitudes.

I get pretty irritated with people who try to climb into the mind of God or ascribe to him a terrible event.

But the inescapable reality is that God is all-powerful, and so he has the unlimited ability to prevent us from being hurt. And he has the ability to make our current pain go away. Often, he does neither.

That can really hurt. It can really slam me to the ground. It often does.

But, when I am rational, I truly believe that God has a reason for what he does, and what he does *not* do. I think I am just too puny to see what he sees, and to know what he has in mind.

Suffering is often a fork in the road that forces people to decide what they believe about God. People who reject God often argue that if he has the ability to relieve human misery and refuses to do so, then he must be a monster. They imagine no other alternatives.

Try explaining to a toddler why Mommy is allowing the doctor to give him a shot in the bum. I don't mean to make light of anyone's pain, and I don't mean to be simplistic. I just want to underscore that there are alternatives to the formula *Existence of Pain = Bad God.*

Saying, "I would do things differently if I were God," is really just a coded way of saying, "I would do things *better* if I were God." It's unbelievably cheeky of me to think that, and I *do* think it sometimes. It means I still have maturing to do.

Does any human really want to assert, "I am kinder, smarter, and morally better than God"? But pain can drive us to think lunatic thoughts.

In sharp contrast, I see mature believers again and again trust that—even if they can't understand a reason for their pain or why God does not relieve it—his *heart* can be trusted. They have confidence in his intent. They are convinced God is good, even if they are suffering. "Though he slay me, yet I will trust in him . . ." (Job 13:15 KJV).

The suffering can be blinding for a while, and bring doubt, confusion, and deep sadness in the soul. But the fog lifts somehow, and they come back to trusting that God is *good*, even if circumstances are terrible and steeped in suffering.

The apostle Paul came to God on three occasions and asked for relief from some painful thing he referred to as a "thorn in the flesh." We don't know what it was. We do know that it hurt, and we also know that God made a specific decision to not relieve the suffering—for reasons he saw and that Paul did not. "My grace is sufficient for you" (2 Cor. 12:1–10 NASB).

The only way I manage any sense of peace when dealing with pain is to settle on the key factor of *intent*. God intends our good. Always. So I have to live with the tension of the unanswered questions.

One of my close friends gave me this advice when I was going through a particularly black time, "Go with what you know instead of probing what you don't know."

That was great counsel.

I don't understand the many hard things that have smashed into my life, or the lives of people I love, but there are a few things I do know with certainty.

Big Thing Number One: Jesus did not shield himself from the pain we experience, but suffered in unspeakably awful ways we will never even begin to touch. And although what was done to Jesus was done by wicked people with dark hearts, God co-opted the evil and brought incredible good from it. God can pull that off. He is that big.

Big Thing Number Two: the Bible asserts that "in all things God works for the good of those who love him, who have been called according to his purpose" (Rom. 8:28). That passage doesn't say *everything is good*. But it does say that "in all things" our Father in heaven is working for our benefit, even if we can't see it. Even in the middle of our pain. He is up to something, and his intent for us is good.

Big Thing Number Three: there is some kind of direct connection between our painful circumstances and our future good. "For our light and momentary troubles are achieving for us an eternal glory that far outweighs them all" (2 Cor. 4:17).

That was penned by someone who, for the sake of Christ, was repeatedly beaten, jailed, persecuted, ostracized, and eventually executed. He was far from glib. He earned the right to say that.

That's really as far as I am comfortable going with this issue. We live in a fallen world, and, even though we all suffer in different ways, the pain is universal. No one gets out of here unscathed. Hey—no one gets out of here alive. The Grim Reaper awaits us all.

But we have a Savior who has likewise suffered. The Son of God actually died, and in the most excruciating way. His pain didn't mean God was aloof or uncaring or sadistic. God was, and is, working for our good. Exhibit A: Jesus rose from the dead after paying for the sin of the world, and he invites anyone who trusts him to spend eternity in a place of spectacular joy.

The pain will end. It will end for your loved one, and it will end for you.

And somehow, although we may not see it, God is with us in the thick of it all. And he is able and willing to extend a supernatural thing called grace to us if we ask for it.

I hope that can bring you a measure of peace, even as life keeps throwing its worst at you.

Let's hang in there, and trust God's intent.

# TWELVE

# The Ebb and Flow
# of Dementia

D
ale and I are continually surprised by what Karin does and doesn't remember. There is no rhyme or reason to it.

Dale came home recently from a visit with her mom and told me, "She has gotten dramatically worse in a week. She used words, but in a way they didn't make sense. She kept saying, 'The children like to lift.' She couldn't have a conversation. I think we may be in that phase where she really can't communicate with us anymore."

With trepidation, we decided to have her over to celebrate Dale's birthday. Our two sons, Mark and Brad, were planning to come over as well. I decided to meet them in the driveway to help them brace for the new reality that their grandmother might not be able to say anything understandable.

Karin had one of her best days in months.

"I'm so glad we can all be together! I think it has been about three weeks since we all saw each other."

"That's about right, Grandma. I've been out of town. Nice to see you again," said Brad, flashing a smile at us.

It was awesome. She went on to talk about all kinds of memories—of farm life, of the kinds of cows they had, how beautiful the flowers were, and so on. We had a great time.

But by the time Dale drove her back to the assisted-living home, Karin was utterly baffled about where she was going, who Dale was, and why she was being dropped off at this brand-new place.

Chalk it up to those neurofibrillary tangles growing in her brain.

She virtually never remembers where she is living. The moment we pull out of her driveway, it's like the place never existed. When we bring her back she will often ask, "Is this where I'm staying tonight? I'll need clothes!"

Sometimes, I will tell her she has clothes in the closet in her room, and she is often mystified by the concept that she has a room in the house.

She can often remember the name of our dog, but have no clue about the identity of lifelong friends.

Our niece JoyAnna lived with us for a semester while she attended a local college. She made the move mostly to spend time with her grandmother. Month after month, she took Karin out shopping, to lunch, and on various excursions. She visited with Karin for hours on end.

"That girl is very nice," Karin said one day. "But I'm not sure who she is, or why she keeps coming over."

In the very early stages of the disease, and before we understood that we could not "help her remember," we would try to fill in the blanks for her. She sometimes covered by saying, "Oh, yes. How silly of me." Maybe sometimes it really did click. But I think that, in many cases, she was simply more puzzled.

"I have grandchildren? No one ever told me."

The clarity factor ebbs and flows.

Sometimes Karin thinks Dale is her mother or her niece or one of her other daughters or simply a vaguely familiar relative. This could happen to you. Just accept that there will be relatively good days and relatively bad days. On her bad days, Karin will demand that we take her home.

*Home* on one of those days can mean Oregon, or the place she lived for decades in Northern California, or Los Angeles, or whatever locale emerges from a random memory.

Because Alzheimer's is so devastating, the diagnosis sometimes sparks denial in family members who simply refuse to admit that a mom, dad, or spouse is in the clutches of the condition.

We know a guy named Scott (not his real name) who was the last holdout in his family. Everyone else believed the diagnosis rendered by a competent physician after a battery of tests. Indeed, it was glaringly obvious to us that Scott's mom had some kind of dementia. You could have an entire conversation with her about a planned outing for the afternoon, and five minutes later she would ask, "So, what are we going to do today?" But for years Scott chalked it up to a natural bit of forgetfulness due to his mom's age.

Then one day, he took her for a long drive. And in the span of a few hours, she asked him what day it was no less than forty times.

Scott reluctantly embraced the reality of what was up with Mom. It wasn't easy. It is never easy. But refusing to accept reality just makes life harder on everyone, especially on the one suffering from the disease. The people who refuse to accept the truth, study up on the condition, and adapt to their loved one are the people you will witness beating the dead horse, frustrated that it won't break into a gallop like it used to. You'll see them accusing it of just being stubborn, convinced that one more whack will do the trick.

Don't be that person.

# THIRTEEN

# Some Can and Do; Some Can't and Shouldn't

It was intended to be a lesson in democracy, but it ended up being more like a tutorial in riot control.

In my former job as an aide to a congressman, I was periodically invited to schools to discuss the principles of representative government. Typically these invitations were at the college level. But one day I received a phone call from a teacher who asked me to address a class of second graders.

Alarm bells started to sound in a tiny little corner of my brain. I mean, it's one thing to engage in a lively debate with a room full of college sophomores. It is quite another to hold the interest of a bunch of seven-year-olds who are far more interested in SpongeBob than the intricacies of modern legislative government.

In the end, I shrugged and asked myself, "How hard can this be?"

(Researchers note that this identical question has been posed by thousands of men shortly before they attempt to replace a faulty electrical socket and subsequently wake up in the emergency room smelling vaguely of singed hair and melted screwdriver.)

And thus I found myself standing before twenty-two grade school children attempting to explain the concept of "majority rules" in voting. I decided that the key to holding their interest was to keep it simple and relevant.

Me: "Let's suppose that we were going to have pie today, but we can only have one kind. Let's take a vote and see how many of you would like apple and how many of you would like cherry."

Little kid: "I want mine with ice cream."

Me: "Well, right now, we're just having a vote on what kind of pie most kids in this room like the best."

Another little kid: "I want mine with milk."

Me: "Let's just hold that thought while we vote."

It was a hotly contested proposition, with passionate arguments on both sides of the issue. But when the votes were cast, the tally came out twelve for apple and ten for cherry. The children were fully engaged, and I felt that the lesson was quite successful.

Me: "And that is how we decide issues in a democratic manner. Any questions?"

Multiple hands shot up.

Little kid: "I want mine warmed in a microwave for twenty-two seconds like my gramma does."

Me: "Well, this was actually just an academic exercise—"

Other little kid: "I want some of each."

Me: "I'm sorry, but perhaps I didn't make it quite clear that this was simply an example of how we decide issues by voting. We are not actually having pie today."

Chorus of little kids: "But you said we were having pie!"

Me (weakly): "Actually, I only posed a theoretical . . ."

Little kid: "They *do* all lie, just like my daddy said!"

The class turned into a festival of denunciations, accusations, recriminations, and pointedly hostile commentary, all directed at the big, fat, cheating liar from the government.

The teacher looked at me with a combination of incredulity at my stupidity and thinly veiled hostility at the mess I had created in her class. I meekly thanked them for their attention and scurried out the door.

God has given us various gifts, and mine are clearly not with kids. My wife, on the other hand, is absolutely amazing with young children. That is why she is an elementary school teacher, and I am not.

Neither of us, though, feel adept at dealing with people with dementia. Honestly, we find it exhausting. We try really hard. Maybe too hard.

"When a conversation hops from one strange subject to another, I get exhausted just trying to figure out something appropriate to say," Dale said to me.

I am in the same boat.

It's hard enough to navigate a conversation with Karin, but it's headache-inducing to try it for more than five minutes with someone we don't really know when we are visiting Karin at her assisted-living home.

But some of the aides we have met seem to thrive on it. They can juggle six Alzheimer's folks at once, moving seamlessly from one "conversation" to another while also filling out charts, administering meds, and escorting someone to the restroom.

If you are wondering how God has gifted you to help others, let me offer this piece of advice: if you can't do it, or if you are utterly terrible at it, it is probably not your calling. If you try taking care of Mom or Dad in your home or theirs, then honestly assess whether you think you have what it takes to be that kind of caregiver. And if riots ensue, as was my case in the classroom, it may not be a good fit.

Our friend Peggy decided to be the caregiver for her mom when that time finally came. She managed to do it for two years, tag teaming with her similarly devoted sister. Her mom eventually moved into the advanced stage of the disease—the kind that requires around-the-clock medical care by nursing staff. Peggy has a great perspective and some really good advice, which I will pretty much just quote for the rest of this chapter.

Thoughts from Peggy:

It is really important to take care of yourself. You are trying to care for someone with a debilitating disease, and you are trying to arm yourself with information and specialists who will help you. And whether you bring Mom or Dad into your own home, or find help to keep them in their own home for as long as possible, or arrange for some type of assisted-care home situation, this is a BIG job. A big job that will only get harder—harder physically, financially, and emotionally.

Caring for someone with Alzheimer's exacts a heavy toll. A Stanford study concluded that Alzheimer's caregivers have a 63 percent higher mortality rate than non-caregivers, and that 40 percent of Alzheimer's caregivers die from stress-related disorders before the patient dies.[1]

This should alert all caregivers that it is not a luxury, but rather an absolute necessity, to care for themselves! They need to find ways to reduce their own stress, eat right, and exercise. It's not just good advice; it could save their life. Stress is a killer in its own right.

And arrange for respite. Do *not* do everything yourself. Get help. Don't hog all the work and worry—learn to share with others! Respite is essential.

My mother was always the sweetest, gentlest, and kindest person I knew, and that remained true all through her years of living with Alzheimer's. Her cognitive and physical condition deteriorated, but her spirit remained loving and generous. Even so, caring for her in my home, although I chose to do it—and would do it again in a heartbeat—took its toll on me.

It was a 24/7 job. I never slept through the night, because I was always listening for her to wake up so that I could make sure she found the bathroom and then make it safely back to her bedroom. I worried about her health, her safety, and her happiness. I loved her unconditionally and with all my heart.

But I needed breaks. If my sister had not lived in town to help out, it would have been so much harder. Even more importantly, since my sister and I were extremely close, we could talk to each other and support each other emotionally. And my husband was my rock. He cared for me every day, and he could tell when I needed a break and made sure it happened.

One day, a close friend of mine from Southern California called and asked me to fly down to visit. She knew I needed a break and thought a weekend on her sailboat would be a quiet and relaxing way to get one. So I did. That first night, she was asleep in her cabin at the end of her thirty-five-foot sailboat, and I was sleeping on a wooden berth under an open hatch next to a slip at the dock. At 2:00 a.m., the owner of a neighboring boat came back drunk and turned up his radio, waking everyone around him, and the other boat owners started yelling at him to turn off his music. My friend woke up, distressed that she had brought me all that way to have a relaxing break only to have all this commotion ensue. She apologized for it in the morning, but I never heard any of it! I—who heard my mother's feet hit the carpeting at the other end of my house every night and became wide awake to watch out for her—never heard any of it, because my brain knew that "I was not responsible." It was okay to relax; I was able to sleep.

In addition to setting up a power of attorney (generally separate ones for financial and medical decisions), make allies of your loved ones' doctors, bankers, etc.

Go with them to their medical appointments so you know what is going on. You can give additional information to the doctors, and you can be able to help with managing their care, medications, etc. It is important to start this process early, while the loved one can still give consent, and you can build a rapport with the doctor. As the condition progresses, the patient may no longer be able to express what is truly happening (or effectively follow a plan of treatment), and if you are not already involved, it is hard to play catch up.

The same is true with bankers or other financial advisors. Get involved early, again while consent can be given. Face-to-face meetings can make the banker your ally as well. You never know when you will have a question or a problem down the road that they can help you solve, just because they know you, trust you, and are willing to go out of their way to help.

I received a check made out to my mother months after she passed away. I had a joint account with her for years and had kept it open for six months after she died, but finally closed it out, thinking there was no point in keeping it open anymore. Right after that I received a check for a few hundred dollars from a large company on the East Coast about a long-forgotten matter. I called them to see if they would reissue it to my name (explaining the situation), and they said I could write a letter to request it, but it likely wouldn't happen. This was very distressing to me. Without much hope, I went to the bank and spoke to a manager who knew me and my mother, and knew we had had a joint account for years. She immediately approved the teller to cash the check—without any further problems—because she knew us.

When I first started taking care of my parents, I needed to make sense of their financial situation and start doing their taxes. (My mother had done it all their lives.) Although their social security and pensions were plenty for them to live on, my mother had also enjoyed buying a variety of stocks over the years . . . which had split, changed names, consolidated, and split again. (Remember the breakup of the Bell System into numerous Baby Bells?) Calculating a basis for these stocks was not a simple matter, but having an ally in the bank and in the bank's financial advisor's office greatly helped me in my research and in selling the stocks when the time came.

Talk with your loved one about what their life was like when they were growing up (or any other topic they want to talk about). It is a chance to engage them in a way they can participate, and you just might learn something. Be patient if they repeat themselves. Consider capturing them on video (or at least recording their voice), no matter what the subject matter. One day, they will no longer be able to speak, and you may wish you could hear their voice again.

Share pictures of them when they were young (if they are interested). It is possible that they will still have memories of that time of their life, even when they no longer are retaining short-term memories of what is happening now. Even if they repeat their stories, listen.

It is important that we enter our loved one's reality, and not try to make them enter ours. Trying to correct them repeatedly only causes them stress and solves nothing.

A friend of mine had her mother living with her who was showing signs of dementia. When her mother started asking where her husband was (who had died more than a decade earlier), at first my friend tried to tell her that he died a long time ago.

"Don't you remember, Mom?"

Of course, her mother did not remember and accused her daughter of keeping it a secret or lying about it. And then she would ask the same question, and it would start all over again. Finally, my friend realized she would have to join her mother's reality. When the question came up again, she replied that Dad was still at work and would be home soon. This satisfied her mother, and dinner continued happily.

The power of music cannot be overemphasized. Playing the "heart" music of your loved one can bring them great joy, not only while they can sing along but also even after they may have lost the ability to speak. If you don't know what their "heart" music is, you can ask other relatives what their favorite tunes were when they were young, or look up what the popular music was when they were growing up.

My sister would always sing with my parents, and even after our mother lost the ability to speak, my sister would still sing "with" her. We could see her lips moving almost imperceptibly at times, so we knew she still knew what was happening. And even when she lost that ability, we sometimes saw a tear form in her eye. Music is powerful; it reaches the soul even when words no longer have any meaning.

If music is the last piece of reality we lose, I think maybe our sense of humor may be our next to last piece. Keep in mind that it may take some detective work to find out what they find funny.

My mother could no longer follow the plotlines of most movies, so they held no enjoyment for her. But one day we put on *The Three Stooges*, and she laughed and laughed . . . and laughed again when we watched it again (it was for the first time as far as she was concerned).

Be aware of possible hazards. Your loved one might not wander outside now, but there will be a first time. Consider door locks (out of reach) and some kind of noisemaker.

My mother once left our house in the middle of the night. We live in the country, and it was pitch black outside. Because we had bells on the door, I heard her go out and immediately ran out after her. She didn't even seem to notice that it was completely dark, or that she was in her nightclothes and walking barefoot on uneven ground. I found her right away and brought her back in no worse for wear, but if I hadn't heard her go out, it could have been a far different story.

Someone said once that dementia is like a movie of your loved one's life, but running backward. It is an apt description. You have a new normal; what they used to be has been lost, but they can do some things. It is natural to lament what they have lost and how hard it is now, but the reality is that they will continue to decline. Instead, try to enjoy what you *do* have; I know it is difficult, but when the inevitable comes and they lose something else, and you have yet another "new" normal, you might find yourself looking back at what you did have and wish you had appreciated it more.

I used to take my mother to lunch. She could no longer read the menus, so after we both looked at them for a few seconds I'd say, "Oh, Mom, they have that spinach salad you enjoy so much. Would you like to order that?" And she could say yes, without having to worry about not knowing how to read the menu or making a choice (when she no longer knew what spinach salad or anything else was). We would mostly eat in silence, except for a bit of small talk I would bring up, since she could no longer carry on any kind of conversation. Although I was happy to have her there with me, I still missed that she couldn't carry on any kind of conversation anymore, and although she dutifully ate her salad, I don't think she could really taste it anymore, as she had already lost her sense of smell. But later, as the disease progressed, and she no longer could even sit up . . . or eat . . . or speak at all, I would have given anything to have lunch with her again.

In addition to caring for her mom with Alzheimer's, Peggy has also been a lifelong caregiver for her son Josh, who was born with cerebral palsy. Peggy herself is a cancer survivor. And that is just the beginning of a list of incredibly difficult things that Peggy and her husband, Greg, have endured over the decades.

I am honored and humbled to know this incredible couple, who have walked through numerous fires and come out the other end with their faith not only intact, but stronger.

I am such a weakling in comparison.

To all of you who serve in a full-time caregiver role for your loved one, you are utterly heroic. And although the world does not know of your sacrifice, God most certainly does. And one day you will hear the deafening roar of angels cheering when God rewards "your work produced by faith, your labor prompted by love, and your endurance inspired by hope in our Lord Jesus Christ" (1 Thess. 1:3).

To those of you who have found that you can't play that role—and Dale and I are in that boat—let me leave you with this story from my youth.

I wouldn't say that my high school algebra teacher hated me, but he definitely did not keep my name on his Christmas card list. Halfway through the semester I raised my hand and asked, "Can we revisit that whole concept of dividing a number by the letter $y$? How does the alphabet have any relationship to math?"

My questions were always a source of great merriment among the rest of the class, but I wasn't being a wise guy. I was being an English major. I understood the complexity of third person perspective and the importance of never allowing my participles to dangle, but I had no clue how to emit a single ounce of algebra.

Mr. Dowse would routinely order me to stay after class so that he could begin a lecture that always began, "Now David, no one can possibly be that stupid, so I have to assume that you're trying to be the class clown."

"But I really am that stupid!" I would protest. "Honest, ask my sister."

At the end of the semester he handed me my grade: a D minus.

"You deserve an F, but I have finally become convinced that you don't have an attitude problem. You have an aptitude problem. I highly suggest that you avoid any occupations that require any use whatsoever of numbers. Stick with English."

It was good advice.

We all have differing abilities. Some people are very gifted craftspeople, but terrible managers. Some people who are great bankers couldn't teach a sixth-grade Sunday school class any more than they could fly a Boeing 747. The Bible speaks of people who have an actual gift of mercy. They are divinely empowered to be compassionate beyond what is normal. I thank God for those people, and confess I am not one of them.

Again, if you are terrible at it, then it is likely not your gift.

But not being gifted is not a Get-Out-of-Caring-for-Free card.

We all have at least a measure of mercy and compassion, and these qualities can grow with use. These are spiritual muscles that need to be exercised to develop.

Find what you actually *can* do, and start by doing that.

Anyone can visit with a loved one, at least for a while.

Anyone with functioning vocal cords can read a story out loud.

If you have an income, you can help out financially.

You can emotionally give *something*. You can be stretched. You can go beyond the comfortable.

If you can't do it all, do what you can. And the angels will cheer for that too.

# FOURTEEN

# And Now a Few Words from Karin's Daughter

I want you to hear directly from my wife, Dale, as she shares with you her perspective as Karin's daughter. I love Karin, but she isn't my mom. And it is just different when the person with Alzheimer's is your parent. We'll do this in a ten question, Q and A format.

*What was your mom like before Alzheimer's moved into her life?*

Independent. Self-reliant. Family oriented. She knew everyone's birthday. She wanted to know what was happening in the world and kept up on the news. She was an RN and had been a nurse right out of college. I looked last week at a pin she received for fifty years of nursing. She would get together with her former classmates, sometimes going on vacation with them.

I read in her old journal recently that she wanted to "get back to my dear patients." She worked in a convalescent hospital, and her patients were important to her.

She was very friendly, always greeting people at church as they walked in the door. She was missions minded and very sincere and devout in her faith. From the time I was very little, my family was supporting orphans in South Korea. Once one orphan grew up, we would start supporting another one. Mom flew to Korea to visit the orphan she was supporting at that time and brought him presents. On the flight home, she helped care for Korean babies who were being adopted and brought home by US parents. She felt like it was a privilege to do that. She had a servant's heart.

*What were the first signs that something was wrong?*

Mail was stacking up on the table, and there were envelopes marked Past Due. My mom had always been very responsible with the bills, so this was out of character. I looked at her checkbook, and it wasn't in any kind of order. My dad at the time had experienced a series of strokes and had dementia, so she was handling everything. It was overwhelming her.

There is nothing like being at your parents' house for long periods of time to really get a sense of what is going on. I could see that things were just not getting done—cleaning and that kind of thing.

And my mom would sometimes admit that she was having trouble with her memory. She would say, "This is disgusting!" when she just couldn't think of a word.

She was starting to say unreasonable things like, "I'm going on vacation," just assuming that my dad would be fine left on his own. And you couldn't talk her through things logically.

*What were your emotions?*

I felt my heart sink. I felt powerless. Sad. Just a very deep sadness that someone who was so capable and independent would be unable to do the things she had done before and still wanted to do.

*What has been the hardest part of this journey?*

When she realized she had a problem, and it was appalling and frightening to her. She said, "This is terrible" and I replied, "We're going to go through this together. You're not going to be alone." It is like when someone gets a cancer diagnosis. You let them know you're going to be with them every step of the way. That is what I have endeavored to do so she wouldn't feel scared and alone.

When they are sensing the loss of their autonomy, they can get frustrated, angry, and embarrassed.

This is kind of strange to say, but it can get kind of easier as the disease progresses. Mom isn't aware of her memory problems now. She isn't that self-aware. But I wish there were more of that fighting spirit that was there in the early stage.

It was also hard to give up defending myself when she would say, "I haven't seen you in years," or "You never have me over to your house." Especially when those statements were completely wrong, and she had just been over yesterday. I had to learn to say, "Well, I'll just have to fix that."

*What have been some bright spots on the way?*

It is a blessing that she has accepted our help. She has never lost her desire to be with our family. In some ways, we are closer than we have ever been before. I am able to do things for her, and she appreciates it. That strengthens a bond.

I have been able to take her for drives into farm country. It is reminiscent of her childhood, and she loves it.

It was a very big event for her when we took her to Oregon and visited her childhood home. She got to visit with some old friends. She knows the person who bought the old family farm, and we were invited to stay in the home. She was almost skipping as we went to the front door.

The way that you (Dave) joke with her, and that she can understand the joke and engage in a repartee, is wonderful. When you ask her if she is going to compliment your "flowing locks," she will roll her eyes and say something like, "Do you mean your *thinning* locks?"

She is generally happy.

*Please talk about the role friends and family have played during this experience.*

The best thing has been conversations with my friend Peggy. Her mom was more advanced in the disease, so I was able to observe Peggy with her mom at her house. Peggy was able to coach me on key things I needed to do, like get my name on Mom's checking account and always go to doctor appointments with her. It was important to have a friend who knew completely what I was talking about when I described the confusion my mom was experiencing. It helped me understand how to navigate things that I would not have otherwise known how to handle. Peggy is the main friend who has walked through this with me.

My other family members—who would have otherwise been more involved on a day-to-day basis—lived hundreds of miles away at the opposite end of the state. Jill and Jonathan (my sister and brother-in-law) and Gene and Lorrie (my brother and sister-in-law) visited when they could and really stepped up financially when Mom needed help. That was huge. They may not be able to be here all the time, but they help with things like legal issues, dealing with the trust, and all kinds of details.

Our kids were also wonderful. Brad spent a lot of time up at Mom's place when she still lived in her own home. He did major amounts of work cleaning up the property; making it firesafe; and getting rid of my dad's "collection" of old cars, buses, motor homes, and all kinds of stuff. Mark was really kind and patient and would visit with Mom for long periods of time. Both of our sons have a big heart for their grandmother.

And you (Dave) have been wonderful. I really appreciate how you have taken care of all kinds of things I don't like to deal with—medical forms, paying her bills, dealing with the DMV, and the thirty car registration notices that showed up in the mail.

*How do you pace yourself?*

You just do the next thing that needs to be done. You try to figure out how to make time to fit in the little things and the big things. Some days you can just do a little thing, like a phone call. If I was working, and just had nothing left at the end of the day, I would not stop by to visit her. The emotional gas tank was empty.

Some people can visit every day like clockwork. I can't. But if we had her over on a Saturday for a nice lunch, and then played corn hole (a beanbag toss game) and looked at photo albums together—that was a nice experience for her, and then I would take a break for the next couple of days.

And we still need to get out on our own. Go out to dinner, even take a vacation.

*What do you do for you—for your own mental health and well-being?*

I keep chocolate around—seriously. Taking walks, getting out in nature is really big for me. I will watch videos of laughing babies or funny dogs. I will watch a favorite TV show—just little stress relievers. Date nights are important. Being able to just go in the kitchen and cook a comforting meal can feel like a little bit of heaven. And, like you (Dave) have told me, "You don't have to be there every day."

It's funny—when I came every day to see her, she would often say, "You never come over. I haven't seen you in months!"

And when I started taking breaks for a few days at a time, she would often say, "You were just here!"

You can't figure it out. You have to do what is realistic for you. The main thing is that they feel loved and cared about.

*What gives you hope?*

Our love for our parents, and our parents' love for us, goes on. It doesn't just dissolve because of death. My mom passed on her faith to me, and I believe we are going to have an eternity in heaven together. The love we have for each other here isn't going to be lost.

*What is your advice to other daughters and sons who are in the same boat as you?*

Just take it a day at a time. Just be there for them. Help them in the way you would want to be helped. I do what I can to make sure my mom feels sheltered from the storm of the illness.

Let your family help. Siblings that you might have thought could not help can totally surprise you. Reach out early to family members and explain what is happening. Talk to them about the practical things that are coming up —things like "we're going to have to get Mom moved."

And help them get educated on the disease. People everywhere are dealing with this, and information and comfort are available to them.

# FIFTEEN

# Practicing without a License

Everything I have written thus far presumes that a competent medical professional has determined that your loved one has Alzheimer's or an irreversible form of dementia. While your personal observations are an important source of information for the doctor, you are in no way capable of rendering a diagnosis unless you have personally been to medical school.

I mentioned earlier that not all dementias are irreversible. But you can't make that determination. Did you know that something as simple as a bladder infection can create mental confusion and disorientation? Or that depression, which is highly treatable, can likewise put someone in a brain fog? Or that someone can suffer something called a transient ischemic attack (TIA), which is a mini stroke that is often a precursor to a big stroke? The symptoms of TIAs come on suddenly and last less than a half hour, but they are just like stroke symptoms. TIAs can include, among other things, sudden trouble speaking or understanding even simple phrases, and impaired ability to walk or just stay balanced.

An infection or immune disorder can look a lot like the stuff you see with dementia, but those conditions can be treatable. A thyroid problem (treatable) or low blood sugar (also treatable) or lack of B-6 and B-12 vitamins (easy to fix) can cause symptoms that mirror dementia.

And let's not forget about brain tumors, exposure to a poison, bad interactions among medications, or even subdural hematoma (bleeding between the brain and the skull that can easily result from a fall). And the list goes on. There are many ways that someone can have highly treatable symptoms that mimic the indicators of irreversible dementia. So by all means, have a doctor determine what is really going on. Don't practice without a license.

The morning after Karin's 911 call and the subsequent late-night visit from a police officer, we took her to the hospital to get completely checked up. Yes, her doctor had already diagnosed her with Alzheimer's. But her confusion had dramatically increased, so we wanted to see if something else was going on that would respond to treatment or a medication. We also had been doing our homework and knew we needed a current assessment before we could place Karin in an assisted-living home—and it was looking more and more likely that was she would be landing there after she got out of the hospital. (Assisted-living facilities often have different kinds of living arrangements and different costs based on the severity of the condition. Some will not take residents with certain needs or behaviors. More on that later.)

We spent several hours in the emergency room while a team of professionals ran a battery of tests to rule out things like infection or TIAs. Once she was medically cleared, she was whisked upstairs and checked into a geriatric mental health ward.

She loved it.

Seriously. She had been a registered nurse all her life, and she believed she had just been called out of retirement.

"I haven't started charting yet, but that will come tomorrow," she whispered to me as they took her to her room.

A psychiatrist spent some time with her, made an assessment, and gave us the scoop.

"Karin is in the moderate to severe stage of the disease," he said. "We could consider a medication called donepezil that can improve the function of nerve cells in the brain. Basically, it helps prevent the breakdown of acetylcholine, which is a chemical that helps the brain with memory and thinking. We find diminished levels of acetylcholine in people who have Alzheimer's. However, it's typically best used in the early stages of the disease. It may not work for her at this point, and there is a possibility it could make things more difficult for her."

"How so?" Dale asked.

"Common side effects can include nausea, vomiting, diarrhea, muscle soreness, insomnia, tiredness, and loss of appetite."

"That sounds awful," I replied.

"And, not often but still possible, it can also make her dizzy or more confused," he added.

"*More* confused? This sounds like the cure is worse than the disease," I said.

"It isn't a cure," he corrected me. "It can simply slow symptoms for awhile. But let's wrap up the other possible side effects."

"There's more?" I asked.

"Lastly, and only rarely, donepezil can cause . . ." (he pulled up a list on his tablet) "bloating, blurred vision, burning or tingling sensations, chills, cough, eye irritation, fever, high or low blood pressure, hives, hot flashes, increased sexual desire, sweating, irregular heartbeat, itching, incontinence, aggression, agitation, delusions, irritability, nervousness, restlessness, tremors, sneezing, increased thirst, nasal congestion, wheezing, and, often redundantly, wrinkled skin. So we would have to see how she responds. Oh, I also understand that she does not have Medicare Part D, so the prescription cost would be out-of-pocket."

He mentioned a brand-name drug and a ballpark price of $800 per month. I almost passed out.

My mind went back more than a decade to when Congress created Prescription Coverage as Part of the Medicare Modernization Act of 2003. The drug benefit went into effect in 2006, and Karin had asked me at the time if I thought it was worth the cost. (I had been working for a member of Congress at the time, so I was quite aware of this new federal program.)

"Absolutely," I told her.

"I think I'll pass," she replied.

"Why?"

"Because I'm healthy, and I don't take any prescriptions," she said.

"But it's highly likely you will as you get older," I said.

"I think I'll be fine," she replied.

"If you don't sign up for it when you're first eligible, it gets progressively more expensive if you decide to sign up later."

"I don't think I'll need it."

At the time, I made a mental note that this decision might become our problem someday. After discussing donepezil, I now wondered if *someday* had become *right now*.

## SIXTEEN

# Paying for All This

After inadvertently terrifying us with the cost of brand-name drugs that might help some of Karin's symptoms, the doctor let us know that drug makers and pharmacies often have special programs and discounts for people who don't have prescription coverage, so we made a note to check into that. But Dale and I were pleasantly surprised to find a chain pharmacy that offered a generic version at about 90 percent less than the name brands for donepezil. Ditto that for her other medications. So we dodged the Rx bullet! Generic medications are your friend, and you should take them out to dinner and send them thank-you cards.

Karin is on two medications consistently, with a couple others thrown in on an "as needed" basis. Her prescription bill is typically between forty and eighty bucks a month. We can handle that. The more daunting cost is for the Festive Acres Assisted-Living Home, which currently runs (pause for a moment while I suck in a huge amount of air) a whopping

$3,700 per month. That cost is subject to change, but it is never change in a downward direction.

It was $3,400 when we started. Yes, we shopped around. According to fairly recent data, the median cost in our home state of California is $3,750. The Genworth 2015 Cost of Care Survey conducted a pretty big sample of nationwide costs, broken down by state. Missouri had the lowest median cost at $2,525, and Washington DC (unsurprisingly) had the highest median price at $7,838.[1] But since the District of Columbia is not a state—and because it is one of the most expensive places in the nation to live—let's consider Alaska as the most expensive state for assisted living, with a median cost of $5,703. The CDC National Survey of Residential Care Facilities also confirms that what we are paying for Karin is a pretty standard cost.[2]

I often get kind of snarky about members of Congress and senators who keep passing gargantuan national budgets with absolutely no plan to get the national debt remotely under control—other than wringing their hands and giving periodic speeches about it, and perhaps secretly hoping a massive meteor crashes into Iowa and wipes us all out before the bill finally comes due. But I need to point out that the federal Medicaid program pays out huge amounts of money for long-term nursing home care for low-income people.

In some states and in some facilities (and under certain rules), Medicaid will also pick up all or some of the costs for assisted living. So the government often pays for exactly the kind of care your loved one needs or may need in the future. I am going to devote a separate chapter to Medicaid (called Medi-Cal in California), because it is a complex program and is also considered the payer of last resort. For years a cottage industry has been devoted to helping people "shield assets," which is a fancy way of saying "shamelessly and deliberately shifting the financial burden to your fellow citizens even when Mom and Dad have resources to meet their own needs."

I believe that is morally wrong. And after getting snookered for decades, state and federal governments are wising up and cracking down. But, like I said, more on Medicaid in another chapter.

Believe me—I have researched how we might get some financial assistance for Karin once her personal resources are exhausted. So I am part of the problem our nation faces by having a debt so large that we have to invent words like *megajillion* because accountants have given up even pretending to understand just how deeply we are in debt. But programs like Medicaid exist, and you should know about them. And, like our national leaders, I am hoping that we will someday run into a friendly leprechaun with a delightful brogue who will lead us to a pot of gold so everything is cool in the end. (That is a far more likely outcome than Congress ever enacting a plan to somewhat slow the inexorable increase in the budget, much less start paying down the national debt.)

In an ideal world, Karin would have a nice stock portfolio and multiple investments in real estate, or even be a member of the British royal family so we could liquidate a few gold brooches or auction off a couple castles to pay for her care. But ours isn't an ideal world.

Dale's parents were honest and hard-working people who had paid off all their debts and got by on social security and a small amount of savings. They probably could have made ends meet until the end of their lives if they had not come down with Alzheimer's (or some other catastrophic illness). In the end, they owned a modest home, a rental property, a small life insurance policy, and an IRA worth about $20,000. They simply did not factor in Alzheimer's disease. And who does?

So by the time she needed assisted living, Karin had enough income and savings to fund only a couple years of care. Seeing that she would burn through her cash in short order, we discussed the issue with Dale's siblings and their spouses. We all swallowed hard and agreed that once Karin's resources ran out, we would split the costs until we could sell off her home and replenish the coffers. And if that money did not last, we agreed to just dig deep and keep funding her care. (Once again, I need to give a big "thank you" to Gene and his wife, Lorrie; Jill and her husband, Jonathan; and Mary Ann for all you have done.)

Once the liquid cash was gone, but before we sold Karin's property, our new cost was akin to taking on an additional house payment. None of us had that kind of extra money coming in each month. And the Ten Commandments specifically rule out knocking off convenience stores (I checked the fine print). But all of us just did what we had to do.

Options included: extra hours at work, dipping into savings, cutting back discretionary expenses, not taking that long-planned vacation, stretching out payments on bills that normally would have been promptly paid off, holding off on a new roof for another year, not replacing a car that was feeling its age, and one of us even resorted to writing a book about the experience. We also redirected some of our charitable giving, because Karin's care was now a top priority. Indeed, it took on the status of a sacred ministry.

"Religion that God our Father accepts as pure and fault-less is this: to look after orphans and widows in their distress and to keep oneself from being polluted by the world" (James 1:27).

Karin is a widow and in distress. She quite literally can't take care of her own needs, so the biblical directive is to "look after" her. When you do that, when you sacrifice time and energy and money for a mom with Alzheimer's disease, you are practicing your religion in a manner that God deems "pure and faultless."

God never said it would be easy. And it isn't. It is a challenge. It sometimes feels like we are just treading water, and someone periodically tosses us an anchor.

"Dear Mrs. Hastings, your health insurance premium is set to rise . . ."

"Hi Dave and Dale, your mom needs additional care, so the monthly fee has to increase . . ."

"The doctor said we need to add a medication . . ."

Glub. Glub. Glub.

If possible, you want to line up the financial resources before you actually need them (presuming there are, indeed, resources available). Finding those resources can become a treasure hunt. If Mom or Dad cannot recall what they have, you need to sift through their filing cabinet or drawers or little hideaway spots for information on insurance policies, mutual funds, annuities, savings accounts, property, and safe-deposit boxes. Is there contact information for a lawyer? Have you found a will?

As we learned when we stumbled across the family trust documents, there can be really important paperwork and information hidden away in a dark corner of a closet (right next to the rather impressive shotgun no one knew was there). Mom and Dad may have assets—and armaments—you never knew existed.

Did Mom and Dad purchase a long-term care policy? Unlikely, but if they did, you have my permission to perform the Ren and Stimpy "Happy Happy Joy Joy" dance. Because it can help a lot. (The policy, I mean. Not the dance. Although, once I think about it, the dance probably can't hurt.)

Karin had a fully paid life insurance policy that we were able to cash in and apply to her housing needs. It was small, about ten grand, but still helpful. The policy was written in such a way that it was easily converted to cash. That isn't always the case.

All life insurance policies aren't the same, and some make it easier or harder to get access to benefits before someone dies. If you find that you can't just cash it out, you may need to check with the life insurance company about "living" or "accelerated" benefits.

There will be a big financial hit when you accelerate benefits. The issuer will often buy back the policy for 50 to 75 percent of its face value, depending on all kinds of ifs, ands, buts, wherefores, provisions, caveats, qualifications, cautions, warnings, conditions, and other lawyerly wordifications all spelled out in tiny print that can't be read without the aid of an electron microscope. But still, it might be ready cash if Mom is in a pinch.

The available cash is going to be based on a combination of factors that include the policy amount, the premiums, and the policyholder's health and age. Some of these policies can't be converted to cash unless the policyholder is terminally ill.

But even with that kind of policy, you still have options. The policy can be sold to a guy named Guido, known to his associates as "The Vampire," for a lump sum that is dramatically lower than the face value of the policy—usually 50 to 75 percent.

Okay, you don't have to actually deal with the mob. It will just kind of feel like it.

Here's how it works. There are "life-settlement" brokers out there, or you can directly contact a "life-settlement" provider. Upon purchasing the policy, the life-settlement company pays the premiums until the policyholder passes away. Then the company gets the money, not the original beneficiaries.

Good-bye, inheritance.

So there are definite downsides to this option.

According to the IRS, "Generally, life insurance proceeds you receive as a beneficiary due to the death of the insured person aren't includable in gross income and you don't have to report them."[3] That's the good news. But getting cash via a life settlement can have tax implications. So you need to be fully informed before you take this step.

But hey, the priority is your loved one. You ultimately need to do what you need to do to take care of Mom or Dad.

Further considerations: your loved one has to give up on privacy. The company will want to see the insurance policy and Mom's medical records, because the offer is going to be based on the policyholder's age and health, the kind of insurance, the premium cost, and the death benefit amount. Basically, the lower the life expectancy and the lower the monthly premium, the more the company will pay for the policy. Yes, this is about wagering on the life expectancy of your loved one. It feels unseemly, and you may feel the need for a few extra showers if you have to do this.

In addition to the possible tax consequences, the sudden influx of cash can impact eligibility for other kinds of help (such as Medicaid). And the people involved in this business can be pushy. Check with your state's department of insurance or other regulatory entity to make sure these people are licensed, and inquire about complaints. Shop around.

In short, it is a tool in the toolbox. It may or may not make sense in your situation.[4]

Another option is a "life assurance" benefit (also known as a "life insurance conversion") that lets Mom transform the life insurance benefit into long-term care payments. Again, expect a big hit on the face amount of the original policy. Life insurance conversion typically pays somewhere between 15 and 50 percent of the policy value. Yikes. But, again, it can be an option in helping you pay for assisted living, especially if there is an acute financial bind.

Which brings me to something called a "bridge loan."

I'm not pitching a particular company, but when I went to the website for Elderlife Financial Services, this huge headline was at the top of the screen: "We help families achieve their long-term plan to pay for senior living by providing our bridge loan to cover short-term costs."[5]

And that is a pretty good summary of a bridge loan.

Scenario: Mom has been living independently in her own home, with kids checking in on her often. But Mom is getting more and more confused, and the family consensus is that she cannot live on her own, so you implement the plan to have her move in with you. There is a room waiting for her, and you have been getting ready for this for a long time. You knew this day would come.

Forty-eight hours later, you are a sleep-deprived zombie, and you just poured Cheerios into the dog's bowl. You had no idea—no idea at all—how enormously difficult this was going to be.

You turn to your spouse and say, "How does she manage to not sleep at night? I think she was up every hour."

Your mate nods and replies, "I accidentally made a peanut butter and mustard sandwich for your lunch. We can't do this. We have to put her in assisted living."

Mom does not have much in the way of savings but does own her home. But it will take time to get it on the market and sold. You can't stay awake for months. You need cash. As in this week. The assisted-living facility will need the first month's rent up front, plus application fees and other costs. You need several thousand dollars at once, and then thousands of dollars each month thereafter.

So you contact a firm like Elderlife that has created a financial product for this very situation. Bridge loans are short-term loans (typically topping out at $50,000) and crafted specifically to finance the move to assisted living or into a continuing-care retirement community (CCRC). And the loan can process as quickly as one day. Seriously. The bridge loan people know what you're up against.

There are two kinds of bridge loans: an unsecured line of credit (higher interest rates will apply, because there is no collateral) or a secured loan (typically, tied to real estate and therefore meriting a lower interest rate).

As the term *bridge* implies, the point of the loan is to get you from one shore to another. To cover a gap. Specifically, this loan is to finance the first several months of living expenses while a home gets sold, other benefits are secured, or other assets are liquidated.

The Elderlife folks note that borrowers have up to five years to repay, but most bridge loans are repaid in less than a year.

Mom or Dad, or their kids, can qualify for both types of loans based on the standard criteria you are probably already used to from applying for a home or car loan. The firm will consider the credit score and credit history of the borrower(s), as well as the debt-to-income ratio. This can be a family affair, with up to six family members cosigning the loan application.

Especially if there is a home that can be sold, a bridge loan can make far more sense than taking a big loss on a life insurance policy purchased by The Vulture and Scrooge Life-Settlement Corporation.

And if your eyes are not already glazing over with financing options, let's talk about annuities.

There is a way in which an annuity is the opposite of an insurance policy. A friend of mine in the insurance industry once told me that "insurance is a gamble in which you bet that something terrible is going to happen to you prematurely and the insurance company bets it won't—and if you win, you lose."

With an annuity, you are betting on living an unusually long life—and if you win, you win! Essentially, you exchange all or part of a nest egg for a predictable monthly payment from the company. Typically, the company will make payments to you for the rest of your life. So once you sign on the dotted line, they have a vested interest in your kicking the bucket as soon as possible. If you purchase an annuity and then the salesperson claims the elevator is not working so you should take the stairs, make him go first.

In addition to an income stream you can count on, the annuity gives you the chance to beat the insurance people at their own game. If you happen to live an unusually long time, you will give a karate chop to the actuarial tables and could end up getting more money from the annuity than you paid into it. That's why an annuity would have been an *awesome* deal for Methuselah.*

Some people hate annuities and think they are a terrible deal. Others view annuities as good options for some people in some situations. Another tool in the financial toolbox. I don't really have a strong opinion either way. But a few cautionary notes are in order.

There are various annuities out there. One will offer a fixed interest rate while another uses a variable rate. Some annuities begin paying you on a future date and some commence payments right away. You'll need to understand what kind of fees are involved. And inflation is not nice to an annuity income. And Guido the Vampire has a kid brother who sells sketchy annuity products and will lie through his teeth. Regrettably, fraud exists in this field of business. Seniors are seen as easy marks. So I suggest getting some advice from a reputable financial adviser.

And just when you thought I was going to move on from mathy subjects, let me introduce the reverse mortgage. This revenue source can make sense when Mom and Dad own their own home (or have it almost paid off), and one of them needs to be moved into assisted living or skilled nursing, but the other partner wishes to keep living in the home.

*He lived 969 years.

(Right off the bat, you need to understand that this option means that the bank plans to eventually sell the house. So if someone in the family is really sentimental about the old homestead, have a box of tissues handy. Or tell them to plan to buy it from the bank.)

The reverse mortgage has the feel of income, but it is basically a loan. The house is the collateral, and the bank sells the house when the occupant passes away. Akin to what can happen with an annuity, if the occupant of the house is unusually healthy and lives to an exceedingly ripe old age, they can end up occupying the house and keep getting monthly payments from the bank, even if the loan balance exceeds the value of the home. *Sweet!*

A reverse mortgage lets Mom or Dad access the value of the home while still living in it. The equity can be taken in a lump sum or in monthly payments. The bank will make an offer based on the value of the home, current interest rates, the age of the person who will continue to live in the home, and a few other considerations. The loan balance is repaid upon the death of the borrower, and that means selling the home to satisfy the loan or cutting a check to the bank for the amount of the loan.

Age restrictions apply, as do some other conditions. But if the borrower is at least sixty-two, this can be a live option.

Let's weigh some pros and cons.

On the plus side, this is ready cash. And even though this is technically a loan, no payments are due unless the occupant sells the home, moves, or passes away. There is the possibility of getting payments that end up exceeding the value of the home (especially likely if you are related to Methuselah). And it is easy to qualify for the loan, because credit score and credit history are not relevant. It is largely about the age of the borrowers and the value of the home.

Most reverse mortgages are administered by the US Department of Housing and Urban Development (HUD), so of course they are not going to call them reverse mortgages. Due to a federal rule requiring that simple words be translated into complicated terms that result in acronyms no one can pronounce, the HUD reverse mortgage program is called the Home Equity Conversion Mortgage (HECM). And before you can receive a reverse mortgage, HUD will require you to speak with a HUD-approved counselor to ensure you know what you are getting into—even though the federal government has found many counselors to be inept. Seriously. I guess it is the thought that counts. But I still have the HUD program in the pro column, because HUD rules stipulate some strong protections for the borrower *and* the heirs.

To quote HUD:

> Once the property is sold—and this can be during the homeowner's lifetime or after his or her death—the sale price of the property pays back the loan. *This rule is in place even if the sale price is less than the combination of the loan and interest (referred to as a short sale)* [emphasis mine]. Because reverse mortgages are backed by HUD, if there is a short sale HUD will pay the difference. Lenders cannot—by law—go after the homeowner's other assets or the estate, so there's no need to worry that your children will have to pay the difference from their inheritance.[6]

That kind of makes up for HUD coming up with the term "HECM."

But what if the reverse is true? What if a lot of value remains in the home? Let's look at a scenario with really easy numbers, because I was a communications major (which is a fancy term for "bad at math").

Suppose that Mom and Dad take out a reverse mortgage on a house appraised at $200,000. And let's say Dad passes away in assisted living while Mom continues living in the home for a few years. Let's say she has received monthly payments that total $100,000, but then also passes away. What happens to the other $100,000 in equity?

No, the bank does not get to just take the money and run. This is not an annuity.

The heirs have some options. They can pay off the balance of the loan and keep the house. Or sell the house, pay off the loan, and pocket the remaining cash. Or let the bank sell the house, and, after the loan is paid off, the remaining equity goes to the estate (the heirs).

The heirs are given six months to deal with paying off the loan. They won't want to dither, because interest will still be accruing on the loan.

On the downside, interest and fees apply. The loan origination fees are unusually high—often double what you would pay for a normal home loan. The loan comes with a variable interest rate. There can be negative impacts on eligibility for state and federal assistance programs (such as Medicaid). And the US Government Accountability Office (GAO) issued a report in 2009 noting that many HUD-approved counselors were making simplistic and misleading statements such as, "This will give you a lifetime income," or "You can't outlive the loan."[7]

Well, this *could* be true, but there are important conditions to those assurances. For instance, the counselors would sometimes neglect to note that monthly payments would not continue if the borrower moved out of the house. They were sloppy, and some of them may still be doing it, even though the GAO gave them all a bit of a chewing out.

You can view the report online (https://www.gao.gov/new.items/d09812t.pdf), and I suggest you do. The misleading statements are detailed, and clarifications are provided.

Karin was not living in her house when we decided to sell it, so the reverse mortgage idea was never even a consideration.

We did, however, sell stuff that was in the house and on the property.

One of our big questions was, "What in the world are all these keys for?"

Dale's dad was a collector, to say the least. He loved vehicles and loved to tinker with them. Roughly thirty vehicles dotted the six acres that he and Karin bought decades ago. And so we faced the question of what to do with a couple dozen passenger cars, two commercial-sized buses, two non-operational motor homes, a couple old Checker cabs, a postal service delivery truck, a vintage Mercedes station wagon, and a World War II–era tractor.

Some were simply projects Dale's dad had never gotten around to, and we had them hauled off for scrap metal. But some were collector's items, and thus assets that could be liquidated. First, though, we had to go through the task of finding buyers.

We did some web searches and found that some of the "junk" was actually in hot demand by people who have way more time on their hands than I do. Wondering if someone just might want the 1960s-era Mercedes station wagon, we had our son Brad post it on Craigslist (because I have the computer and technical skills of an Amish grandmother). It took about ninety seconds for someone to call him.

"I'll take it. I'm driving up tomorrow."

Brad pointed out that the vehicle was rusty, not working, and sitting on rims.

"Perfect. How much do you want for it?"

"How about, uh, $1,800?"

"Deal."

One man's trash is another man's answer to a lifelong quest for the perfect project.

When we got the property about as cleared as possible, we prepared to put it on the market "as-is." That meant whoever wanted to buy the home (which, honestly, had seen better days) also needed to be prepared to own a few buses and other vehicular objects in various states of disrepair, a chicken coop, a goat pen, a massive light that was once part of an airport, all manner of tools and screws and metal bits of random stuff collected over the past several decades, and every single copy of *National Geographic* published since the Kennedy administration.

Dale's brother, Gene, did the legwork on the real estate front. Several agents listened to the description of the property and turned Gene's business down flat. They were too professional to break into unbridled gales of mirth and double over trying to catch their breath, but we all got the point. This was going to be tough to sell.

Gene finally stumbled onto an eager agent named John, who loved a challenge. He felt he could sell it in a timely manner. I, on the other hand, suspected we would be waiting until the return of Halley's comet. For the record, that's in the year 2062.

We had an offer within a few weeks.

"They're offering almost the asking price," the agent said.

"Are they clear on the fact that we're not going to tidy up the property any more than we already have, and that we're not hauling off any of the cars or tractor discs or otherwise-enormous objects?"

"Oh, yes. In fact, they stipulated that they want everything that's on the parcel as of today. They want it all."

"So, you're telling me they're insane?" I replied.

"Some people love stuff," he said.

We closed, banked the money, and used it for Karin's care.

Besides looking for obvious assets like bank accounts, IRAs, jewelry, real estate, and other valuables, you should look at programs that may apply. If your loved one is a veteran, you should check with the Department of Veterans Affairs (VA) about available assistance.[8]

A veteran *may* be eligible for help with assisted living, residential (live-in) care, or home health care. I say "may," because the VA considers a host of factors that range from your income to whether you have a service-connected disability (a disability that resulted from military service). And if your loved one happens to have received the Medal of Honor, they are going to be treated like royalty and likely go to the head of the line for placement in a State Veterans Home (more on the State Homes in a bit).

The VA website notes that, in addition to standard health care, VA services can include:

24/7 nursing and medical care, physical therapy, help with daily tasks (like bathing, dressing, making meals, and taking medicine), comfort care and help with managing pain, and support for caregivers who may need skilled help or a break so they can work, travel, or run errands.

Veterans can get this care in many different settings. Some are run by VA and others are run by state or community organizations that the VA inspects and approves, including: nursing homes, assisted-living centers, private homes where a caregiver supports a small group of individuals, adult day health centers, and the veterans' own homes.

You may be able to use one or more of these services if: you're signed up for VA health care, and the VA concludes that you need a specific service to help with ongoing treatment and personal care, and the service (or space in the care setting) is available near you.[9]

If your loved one is not already enrolled in the VA health care program, you can help them apply for benefits. They earned it by serving the nation.

My city is home to a State Veterans Home, which is a state-run facility that provides full-time care for veterans and, in some cases, their nonveteran spouse and even Gold Star parents (parents who have lost a child due to service in the armed forces). There are more than 150 State Veterans Homes in the US. Many have a special section to meet the needs of dementia patients.

The veterans home in my town is awesome. Beautiful grounds, nice rooms, good food, caring staff, and round-the-clock care. These homes are partnerships in which the federal government shares the cost of building and operating the home, but the facility is owned, staffed, and managed by the state. (I was privileged, as a congressional aide, to play a smidge of a role in my hometown project. It makes me happy every time I drive by it.)

The VA can be of enormous help in keeping your veteran loved one at home as long as possible. They have home-based primary care where a VA health care team comes to the veteran to provide a wide range of medical services (including help with daily tasks). The VA can also provide a home-maker/home health aide (supervised by a registered nurse) who comes into the veteran's home to help with self-care.

The VA even features something called "adult day care" where a veteran can go during the day for social activities, companionship, and recreation, in addition to health care. The VA can also provide in-home palliative (pain management) care and hospice (end-of-life care, covered in-depth in a later chapter).

The VA notes that "the United States has the most comprehensive system of assistance for Veterans of any nation in the world, with roots that can be traced back to 1636, when the Pilgrims of Plymouth Colony were at war with the Pequot Indians. The Pilgrims passed a law that stated that disabled soldiers would be supported by the colony."[10]

I think the Pilgrims would approve of the range of services offered to veterans today. So, if Mom or Dad served in the armed forces of the United States, by all means see if the VA can help in this time of need.

# SEVENTEEN

# Medicare and Medicaid— How They Will and Won't Help

Geneal rule:
Medicare *does not* pay for long-term care or assisted living.

Medicaid *often* pays for long-term care and assisted living.

But a boatload of caveats has now pulled up to the dock, and we need to commence unloading them. By the time we are done unpacking and stacking all the rules, qualifications, waivers, eligibility criteria, and all manner of other guidelines, you will need an adult beverage on the rocks or a glass of warm milk and a nap.

I was tempted to shorten this chapter to this one sentence: "Check with your county social service office to see if your loved one qualifies for help with in-home care, long-term care, or assisted living." That is because Medicaid is a state and federal partnership, and one size does not fit all.

Different states have their own variations in the Medicaid program.

Medicaid has become such a complex program that the US Department of Health and Human Services included this sentence in a report: "Medicaid now offers so many options for providing home and community services that they can be confusing for policymakers, state officials, advocates, and consumers alike."[1]

Yes, your government finds its *own program* to be baffling. However, they do wish you well as you seek to sort it all out.

California doesn't even call it Medicaid, because years ago someone decided it would be extremely clever to call it something else.

Stan: "Hey Norm, let's get the California legislature to rename the Medicaid program Medi-Cal!"

Norm: "Why?"

Stan: "Look how *ingenious* it is to combine 'medical' and 'California!' You get *Medi-Cal*. Get it? Get it? No other state can do this! Connecticut would end up with 'Medi-Con' and North Dakota would be 'Medi-No.' We're *unique* in being able to do this!"

Norm: "Won't that just confuse the people who are trying to sign up for it?"

Stan: "That's beside the point. This is about being adroit with the English language."

Norm: "But we'll have to change a ton of forms, brochures, signs, phone listings, decals, letterheads, and that kind of thing. It'll cost a fortune and be a paperwork nightmare, and it's completely unnecessary."

Stan: "We'll probably have to hire a new army of bureaucrats to implement it. Our department will grow overnight."

Norm: "Why didn't you say so to begin with? Awesome idea, Stan!"

I refuse to play along with this silliness, so if you live in California, just understand that I am including Medi-Cal when I discuss Medicaid.

Let's first review the broad differences between Medicare and Medicaid.

The first big difference is that, generally speaking, Medicare is age-based and Medicaid is income-based.

Warren Buffet is so rich he can purchase the entire state of Nebraska (and may have already done so), but he qualifies for Medicare. Bill Gates is worth somewhere in the vicinity of $85 billion, and it is therefore unlikely that he struggles to pay for an annual prostate exam. Doesn't matter. The minute he turns sixty-five, he is eligible for Medicare. Indeed, he will have to fill out a form specifically asking *not* to be enrolled in at least one part of Medicare if he wants to decline coverage. (And that would be a nice gesture of him.) But Bill Gates and Warren Buffet will *never* qualify for Medicaid, because they will never be poor.

If your loved one is sixty-five or older, a US citizen, and paid into social security and Medicare for at least ten years or was married to someone who did so, they qualify for Medicare coverage. (You can also qualify for Medicare if you become disabled before you turn sixty-five, but a two-year waiting period applies for most people.) Legal, permanent residents who are not citizens can also qualify, but other rules apply (such as the "five consecutive years residency" requirement), so they need to check with Medicare.

Medicare is divided into several parts.

Part A covers hospitalization, and that coverage comes at no charge. (And that, dear reader, helps explain our enormous national debt. Congress is really good at giving things away, but very hazy on a concept known as "math.")

Part B covers many (but not all) doctors' services, outpatient care, medical supplies, and preventive services, but you have to sign up for it and pay the monthly premium that is north of one hundred dollars and subject to change (but, like assisted-living costs, the change is always in an upward direction).

Part C is a "Medicare Advantage Plan." If Mom or Dad selects this option, a private company has a contract with Medicare to provide both Part A and Part B benefits—and usually prescription drug coverage as well.

Part D is prescription drug coverage. The premium will vary by what plan you choose and your income level. Part D also has something called a "donut hole," a term used to describe a temporary gap in coverage. The coverage gap is a design feature, not a bug. (Congress finally started to sort of understand the math and used a cost-saving formula that no one on the planet completely fathoms.)

To help "clarify" the implications of the coverage gap, the Medicare website features this information:

Not everyone will enter the coverage gap. The coverage gap begins after you and your drug plan have spent a certain amount for covered drugs. In 2017, once you and your plan have spent $3,700 on covered drugs, you're in the coverage gap. This amount may change each year. Also, people with Medicare who get Extra Help paying Part D costs won't enter the coverage gap.

The website then provides this example:

> In 2018, Mrs. Anderson reaches the coverage gap in her Medicare drug plan. She goes to her pharmacy to fill a prescription for a covered brand-name drug. The price for the drug is $60, and there's a $2 dispensing fee that gets added to the cost. Mrs. Anderson pays 40% of the plan's cost for the drug and dispensing fee ($62 x .40 = $24.80).
>
> The amount Mrs. Anderson pays ($24.80) plus the manufacturer discount payment ($30.00) count as out-of-pocket spending. So, $54.80 counts as out-of-pocket spending and helps Mrs. Anderson get out of the coverage gap. The remaining $7.20, which is 10% of the drug cost and 60% of the dispensing fee paid by the drug plan, doesn't count toward Mrs. Anderson's out-of-pocket spending.[2]

After reading this example, Mrs. Anderson will likely pop a few Xanax and just hurl random amounts of cash at the pharmacy clerk.

None of those parts of Medicare pay for assisted living or nonmedical, long-term care.

But Medicare *can* cover a "medically necessary" short-term stay in somewhere that is less than a hospital, and that is also chock-full of people who are on Medicaid for a long-term stay.

Medicare looks at a skilled-nursing facility room and says, "Don't start hanging pictures on the wall; you won't be here long. And get ready for some copayments."

Medicaid looks at that same room and says, "Welcome to your new home. It's on the house."

Like I said, these are very different programs.

According to the Medicare.gov website, "Medicare Part A (Hospital Insurance) covers skilled nursing care provided in a skilled nursing facility (SNF) under certain conditions for a limited time. Medicare-covered services include, but aren't limited to:

Semi-private room (a room you share with other patients)
Meals
Skilled nursing care
Physical and occupational therapy (if they're needed to meet your health goal)
Speech-language pathology services (if they're needed to meet your health goal)
Medical social services
Medications
Medical supplies and equipment used in the facility
Ambulance transportation (when other transportation endangers health) to the nearest supplier of needed services that aren't available at the SNF
Dietary counseling"[3]

Basically, Medicare will cover short-term care following a medically necessary three-day stay in the hospital. They count the day you get admitted, but not the day you are discharged. A hundred-day clock is ticking on a hospital/ skilled-nursing facility stay. Medicare requires you to foot the bill for any days after the one hundred mark.

Let's say Mom or Dad gets hospitalized (for at least three days) and then needs time in a skilled-nursing or rehabilitation facility to recover from injury, illness, or surgery. Part A can do that. If Mom's stay is between one and twenty days, Part A picks up the tab (minus her deductible). From days twenty-one to one hundred, Mom has to kick in a daily coinsurance. If she has a Medicare supplement policy, that policy will likely cover it (depending on the plan she purchased). After one hundred days, Part A coverage vanishes. She can stay in the facility, but at her own cost. That one hundred-day stay is called a "benefit period." Sixty "healthy" days must elapse before Mom is eligible for a new "benefit period." (No runs to the emergency room, for example.) There is no limit to how many sets of one hundred-day hospital coverage days can be used as long as the intervening sixty-day period keeps getting met.

Since most people do not schedule their illnesses in order to meet the Medicare criteria, the required conditions for a covered hospital stay can seem irrational to a normal person. If you find yourself bewildered by this collection of seemingly random and odd rules, congratulations—you are in the population of normal people. If any of this makes sense to you, then you probably work for Medicare and you have gotten used to it. I hope for your eventual return to the realms of normalcy.

Medicare will not kick in for "custodial" (nonmedical) residential care in either a nursing home or assisted-living facility. Having dementia and being confused and unable to take care of yourself is not considered a "medical" condition for the purposes of Medicare coverage. But it is a covered condition under Medicaid.

So Medicaid routinely covers long-term medical *and* custodial care and *may* cover nonmedical residential care—what you and I call assisted living. It depends on a host of factors. (And when I say "long-term" I mean "for the rest of their life, if need be.") Unlike Medicare, Medicaid does not have a clock ticking on its coverage.

Medicare is a defined benefit, and payments to providers are comparatively generous. Medicaid pays on an open-ended basis, even for the rest of your life, but often at a bargain basement rate (which is why a lot of doctors and facilities refuse to participate in the Medicaid program). Basically, a person does not qualify for Medicaid until he is broke. And that is as it should be, in my humble opinion.

The government expects you to burn through your own resources before turning to the Medicaid program, because the term "Medicaid" is just a euphemism for "my fellow taxpayers."

The Medicaid money does not come from thin air. Like many government programs; Medicaid simply transfers money from one set of taxpayers to another. It is eminently reasonable to require the use of personal resources as the primary way to meet personal needs.

We have liquidated, or are in the process of liquidating, every asset we can find that Gene and Karin owned. We are aware that this means there will not be anything to inherit. And that is okay. Karin's stuff should be used for Karin. Only after all those resources are exhausted would we feel decent about seeking help from the government safety net.

There has long been a "Medicaid Planning" industry staffed by clever people with green eyeshades who will use every trick in the book to legally "shield your assets" so you can use public loot instead of your own. A favorite scheme is to start transferring money to family members years before you think you may "need" Medicaid. People hire attorneys to help them plan to become "impoverished" enough to qualify for public assistance.

I think this reeks.

Medicaid was intended to be a payer of last resort. More than a decade ago the *Wall Street Journal* ran a story called "Medicaid for Millionaires." The headline alone tells you that something has gone horribly awry.

The *Journal* piece begins thus:

> Medicaid was established in 1965 with the worthy aim of providing medical care for the poor; it was never intended as a middle-class entitlement or as inheritance protection for the children of well-off seniors. Yet the latter is precisely what has happened—to the point that sheltering assets and income to qualify for Medicaid is now as routine as writing a will.[4]

The government is trying to catch up, and there are now "look back" and "claw back" provisions that allow the recovery of "gifted assets" when the gift giver then seeks Medicaid services.

I could quote you stuff about annual income and asset tests, but this stuff is subject to change and I don't want to lock in stale information. Congress has spent years considering major changes to Medicaid, because the costs are exploding every year. Anything I write on this subject today could be old news by tomorrow.

But as of the date of this writing, the Medicaid program pays for skilled-nursing care in all fifty states. Additionally, as noted earlier, in *some* states and in *some* participating facilities, Medicaid can pay for assisted living. Basically, the government decided that if someone would be eligible for care in a skilled-nursing facility (which is extremely expensive) but can actually have their needs met in assisted living (not nearly as expensive), it just makes fiscal sense to pay for assisted living.

This is one of those happy occasions when the government spends money like a normal person instead of an entity that is smug because it can print its own currency.

I can't list the places where the government will pay for assisted living. The program is subject to change, states can change their rules, and facilities can opt in or out. So you need to contact your local Medicaid administrative office (typically a department in your county government). Often, a facility will only have a limited number of "Medicaid beds" because the reimbursement is not as high as they want it to be (but I think it is still *plenty* high). The median cost per month in California tops $7,000 per month for a shared room in a skilled-nursing facility. The median monthly cost in Alaska is more than $20,000 for skilled nursing. Bear in mind, this is not for hospital level care. This is what is commonly known as nursing home care.[5]

While the federal government picks up most of the tab for a stay in a Medicaid-approved facility, there is still an expectation of a copayment.

Let's say Dad is approved for a "Medicaid bed." His social security check is pretty much going to have to be signed over to the facility. The check will still come to him, but he needs to turn over most of the proceeds as the "patient pay" amount. He will be able to keep a nominal amount for personal needs.

If Dad is paying for supplemental health insurance (as is typical for most seniors), he can still pay that out of his social security check before handing over the remainder to the facility. Ditto that for prescriptions and vision and dental insurance, if he happens to also have those. If Dad cancels that other coverage thinking he will then have more personal spending money, he is wrong. The "saved" money will just go to the nursing home or assisted-living facility. He is only going to get the sixty or so bucks that is allowed for personal expenses.

When I said you have to be broke to qualify for Medicaid, I meant it.

To qualify, you can currently only have $2,000 in cash.

But there is a big loophole to the "you must be broke" rule. And that is your home. Unless you live in a mansion, the value of your home (up to a half a million bucks) is not counted as an asset for the purposes of *qualifying* for Medicaid. I have no idea why. I mean, that is a huge asset the way any regular person would count an asset. Some states even exclude a home value up to $750,000.

But don't get too giddy. While the government may not count your home as an asset while you are living, they often take quite a different point of view once you die (this varies by state). It is called cost recovery.

Here is a note from the state of California (in answer to the question, "If I sign up for Medi-Cal, will anything happen to my assets?"):

Medi-Cal only tries to recover its costs for medical assistance after your death when a recipient is over age 55, or when a member of any age is cared for at an institution, such as a nursing home. Medi-Cal does not seek payment during your lifetime or the lifetimes of your surviving spouse, disabled son or daughter, or while your child is under 21 years of age. If you are under 55, you can sign up for Medi-Cal knowing that nothing will happen to your assets unless you are institutionalized. For those over age 55 or in an institution, the

Department of Health Care Services may present a claim for the cost of your care. It would be paid from your estate at the time of your death.*[6]

The state can be patient, but they plan to get as much from you as possible somewhere down the road. If a deceased person owns nothing when they die, nothing will be owed.

Again, an industry out there is dedicated to using every legal tool available to keep the government at bay after you pass away. But just be aware that, depending on the rules in effect where you live, they may come after the value of your home and other stuff you owned that has value. Just putting all your possessions in a "trust" does not deprive the state of the ability to get assets. There may be lawful ways for stuff to be transferred out of your name, but I am not an attorney or estate planner, and I am not going to get into that. You already know my personal opinion on this.

Other exemptions to the Medicaid "you must be broke to qualify" rule:

**A car.** There used to be a requirement that only a modest vehicle that was worth $4,500 or less could be exempted. Currently, there is no cap on the value of a car.

**Prepaid burial plans.** The value of that plan is excluded, even if the plan includes your entire family and you

*Due to Senate Bill 833, California has updated its rules for Medi-Cal recipients who die on or after January 1, 2017. Repayment will be limited only to estate assets subject to probate that were owned by the deceased member at the time of death. For Medi-Cal recipients who die prior to January 1, 2017, repayment will be sought from all assets owned by the deceased member at the time of death. I will not attempt to explain these differences, any more than I would attempt to interpret ancient Egyptian hieroglyphics.

have fourteen kids. Or, if you have a designated bank account to deal with burial arrangements, you can exclude up to $1,500. Ask your bank and they can probably tell you how to set it up, or check with the county Medicaid folks.

**Term life insurance.** Because there is no "cash value" to term insurance, it isn't counted against you. But if your policy has a cash value, that can be counted.

**Oodles of other apparently random stuff.** The huge and complicated list can be found on the Social Security Administration's website.

According to the Social Security Administration, all kinds of things are also excluded when determining your resources. The list includes stuff like: "Stock in regional or village corporations held by natives of Alaska during the twenty-year period in which the stock is inalienable pursuant to the Alaska Native Claims Settlement Act (see § 416.1228)" and "Disaster relief assistance as provided in § 416.1237" and "Restitution of title II, title VIII or title XVI benefits because of misuse by certain representative payees as provided in § 416.1249."[7]

Most of the list is "eyes glaze over" stuff that has narrow application. But you might want to check out the list to see if the shoe fits.

While a person needs to overcome many hurdles before qualifying for Medicaid, millions of people are in the program. Indeed, the *majority* of people in skilled-nursing facilities are funded by Medicaid. So qualifying is certainly not impossible. And, as noted in a prior chapter, about 40 percent of assisted-living facilities had one or more residents who had some or all of their long-term care services paid by Medicaid. So those places are out there if you look hard enough.

Private pay in an assisted-living facility is obviously a costly option, but it also often means a better living environment for the patient/resident. If a non-Medicaid funding source is available for Mom or Dad, they can often have a better quality of life. If Medicaid is a financial necessity, then do your homework and find the best place you can. Not all Medicaid beds are equal. We have all read those stories about dreadful nursing homes being fined or shut down because they were treating their patients atrociously. You really need to have your eyes on the place before allowing Mom or Dad to be placed there.

I would be remiss if I did not point out that both Medicare and Medicaid have a variety of services that can be provided in the home if Mom or Dad does not need a 24/7 skilled-nursing facility. But, again, those kinds of services have different eligibility criteria. And what Medicare pays for will have a limit on the duration.

I want to end on a positive note, so let me break some good news to you: most states allow certain family members to be paid by Medicaid for providing personal care to Medicaid-eligible loved ones living in a home. This does not have to be "medical" care.

Medicaid can pay you for the kinds of normal stuff that needs to be done, but that Mom or Dad can't do on their own. This can include cooking and cleaning, assistance with bathing and mobility, grocery shopping, and doing the laundry.

Because it is waaaaaaaay cheaper to keep Mom or Dad at home as opposed to either assisted living or skilled nursing, Medicaid can even kick in for things like vehicle modifications, stair lifts, wheelchair ramps, and walk-in bathtubs. A wide variety of supplies and equipment can be covered by Medicaid as long as the stuff is medically necessary. And, lest you get overwhelmed by caregiving, Medicaid has been known to cover respite care to give you a break.

All of this can be a huge benefit to a son or daughter who can't afford to give up a job but feels compelled to try and be there for Mom or Dad.

Here is how it works.

Mom (who is broke) applies for Medicaid and gets approved. Mom then applies for and receives a Medicaid waiver that pays for home care and also permits "Consumer Direction." Consumer Direction is government-speak for "Mom can pick her care provider instead of having Medicaid make the choice for her."

Bam! You are now *employed* to take care of Mom. You submit a time card and get reimbursed for your services (but your hours and services will be determined by relevant rules based on what Mom or Dad is deemed to need).

One big caveat before you start celebrating this news: Medicaid prohibits caregiver payment to legal guardians and spouses. And, just because this is a government program and therefore it has to contain at least one bizarre feature, Medicaid will happily pay a *former* spouse to be a caregiver. So if Mom is in a loving relationship with her current husband, tough luck for him on the financial front. But if the guy she divorced and can't stand wants to help out, he is eligible for the Employee of the Month award.

I am going to end this chapter before I go on another rant.

(Official disclaimer: Dave is not a financial planner or anything that would be remotely considered an expert in anything that involves numbers. Dave has not balanced his checkbook since the Carter administration. He just keeps a huge "overdraft line of credit" on his account and pays it off when he inadvertently dips into a negative balance. Dave is also not an attorney, which should surprise no one. He has done the best he can to convey the facts as he understands them, but you need to perform your own due diligence or consult real experts when making big honking financial and legal decisions. Dave will now stop writing about himself in the third person, because it seems kind of weird.)

# EIGHTEEN

# Are You Smoking Something?

A medical research report titled "Amyloid Proteotoxicity Initiates an Inflammatory Response Blocked
by Cannabinoids" was published in the 2016 online version of *Nature Partner Journals*: *Aging and Mechanisms of Disease*.

It included lots of paragraphs like this one:

The above data show that Aβ accumulation in a human CNS
nerve cell line leads to the synthesis of proinflammatory
cytokines and chemokines, elevated eicosanoid synthesis
and the activation of inflammatory pathways. Prostaglan-
dins tend to be neuroprotective and leukotrienes potentiate
toxicity, whereas the activation of cannabinoid receptors
prevents Aβ accumulation and toxicity. Both intracellular
Aβ accumulation and nerve cell death are potentiated by
5-LOX metabolites and proinflammatory cytokines.[1]

This is an extremely scientific and highly wordified way of saying that marijuana (specifically the psychoactive ingredient of marijuana, THC [tetrahydrocannabinol]) might help fight Alzheimer's disease.

Do *not* leap to any conclusions here, and under no circumstances should you decide to experiment on Grandma. The researchers published some interesting findings that need to be subjected to all kinds of rigorous peer review, testing, and a bazillion protocols and permissions and probably even congressional hearings and shouting matches before the Food and Drug Administration (FDA) even remotely considers the possibility of a THC product for human use. A lot of very mellow and unmotivated laboratory rats stand between this early research and any practical use in humans.

I just want you to be aware that the study found that THC stimulates the removal of toxic plaque in the brain. Plaque is a common feature in the brains of people who suffer from Alzheimer's disease. The researchers also found that THC blocks inflammation in the brain. Inflammation plays havoc with neurons and therefore havoc with memory and the processing of information.

David Schubert, a senior researcher and professor at the prestigious Salk Institute for Biological Studies, said, "It is reasonable to conclude that there is a therapeutic potential of cannabinoids for the treatment of Alzheimer's disease."[2]

Note that he says there is *potential*. He doesn't say, "Bake Mom some pot brownies," or "Roll a joint for Uncle Fred." Likewise, Keith Fargo, the director of scientific programs and outreach for the Alzheimer's Association, says that marijuana is a "legitimate avenue of research."[3] The operative term is "research," not "experimentation by concerned family members who have decided to just wing it and hope Grandma does not start seeing purple unicorns."

I know it can be frustrating to wait for years of research followed by more years of meticulous review by the very cautious and anal-retentive FDA. But these processes exist precisely to employ the kind of scientific rigor that moved us beyond the days when people poured mercury on wounds or rubbed chopped mice on warts (this was quite popular in Ye Olde England, which I say is yet one more reason America was right to revolt against Britain).[4]

I know that for some of my more conservative readers the very notion of a benefit from marijuana can seem scandalous, which is why I want to shift to the somewhat safer subject of the possible benefits of cigarettes. Well, not of cigarettes, but of nicotine.

For a few decades, researchers at the Georgetown University Medical Center worked on a study showing that nicotine patches improve mild cognitive impairment (MCI) in older adults. Findings were published in 2012 in the journal *Neurology*.[5] Three academic medical centers took part in the study, which demonstrated that patients who used nicotine patches for six months regained up to (drum roll please) an impressive 46 percent of normal performance (for their age group) on some long-term memory tests. A placebo group got *worse* by 26 percent during the same time frame.

So, just how does nicotine help improve brain function for people with MCI?

Well, your brain has something called nicotinic acetylcholine receptors (don't even try to pronounce it). People with Alzheimer's disease experience a big loss of those receptors, which are stimulated by nicotine and acetylcholine (a neurotransmitter, for those of you who, like me, barely passed biology in high school).

I know, I know. Who would have thought that nicotine could possibly have a benefit? I will confess that I am a reflexively conservative person with a lifelong bias against pot, cigarettes, and that lousy music that blasts from the car of the kid down the street. So it feels weird to be discussing the bright side of THC and nicotine. But we need to just let the facts drive this issue.

Smoking cigarettes is categorically terrible for you, so if Aunt Jenny is showing some early signs of confusion or impaired memory, please do not buy her a pack of Marlboros to get nicotine into her system. And ditto for nicotine patches, unless her doctor is on board. Nicotine is addictive, and its use should not be taken lightly. But the potential benefits of nicotine (without the smoke) are intriguing, at least for the early stages of the disease we have all come to loathe.

"We may have some early evidence that could suggest nicotine can change the course of MCI, and possibly slow progression to Alzheimer's disease," according to Ken Kellar, professor of pharmacology and a member of the Georgetown University Medical Center team of researchers.[6]

(By the way, in an effort to make the study unbiased and fairly bulletproof, the study was conducted "blind." In research-speak, this means that neither the researchers nor the subjects knew who got the nicotine and who got the placebo.)

While the researchers were heartened by the results, they cautioned that the findings do not mean this is a suitable treatment for all people with MCI. The results are a reason for more study, including whether the benefits are long term. But, again, it seems very promising.

I only hope that ongoing scientific inquiry does not raise the inkling of any possible beneficial effect of obnoxiously loud and incoherent music. I can only take so much.

# NINETEEN

# Am I Wasting My Time?

Dale regularly takes her mom on a drive in the rural parts of our community because Karin was raised on a farm and loves to see cows and horses. By the time Dale pulls back into the driveway, Karin has often completely forgotten that they went anywhere or saw anything.

So, was it a waste of time?

Not at all.

Because, while they were seeing the animals, Karin was having a wonderful time.

"Look at all those cows. We had Jerseys. And look at that Palomino! What a beautiful horse!"

She will comment on the trees, the color of the sky, the startling profusion of roses in front of a certain house.

So much of navigating Alzheimer's is about living in the moment. If your loved one can have joy in the immediate present, that is wonderful. Enjoy it with them while they still have the capacity for little pleasures of life.

Yes, it can be disappointing to cook a wonderful holiday meal and have a nice evening with Mom or Dad, and then have them ask you two hours later when the turkey will be ready. But it wasn't a waste. You had the meal together, and that is a success. It is now a memory for you, even if it isn't a memory for them.

Having Mom join you for a meal, even if she forgets it in a few minutes, is infinitely better than having Mom bedridden and unable to speak.

Moments.

Enjoy those moments when you can still bring her a smile, when she can enjoy the Christmas tree, when she can give you a hug good night. Things are going to get worse, not better. You have to make the most of what you still have.

A big part of how well you navigate hard things in life—whether disease or some other kind of heartache—is going to be determined by what you choose to dwell on. I learned that lesson forcefully when I met Captain Brien Thomas Collins back in 1992.

BT, as he liked to be called, was a Green Beret on his second tour of duty when a grenade exploded, shredding his body and nearly costing him his life. Years later he was at a Fourth of July picnic telling a small group of us about the event that forever changed his life.

"So I lost an arm and a leg in Vietnam," he said, motioning with the metal hook that served as his hand. Then he flashed a smile and continued, "But I still had an arm and a leg."

The two sets of facts were equally true. But BT decided to focus on what he still possessed instead of what he had lost. And that choice defined what kind of life he would choose to have. It also shaped the message he would take to his wounded comrades: you can spend your life angry and bitter about what has happened, or you can go on from here and make a life worth living. Choose.

After the blast that mangled his body, BT spent twenty-two months in seven military hospitals as doctors pieced him back together and remedied his numerous complications. But when he got wind of a soldier who had lost a hand or an eye or suffered some other grievous injury, he would cancel his own medical appointment and head to where that soldier was—sometimes driving for hours to meet a wounded warrior he didn't even know.

It was one thing for a completely healthy doctor to tell an amputee that he could still have a good life. It was quite another to hear that message from Captain Collins.

All of us have wounds, losses, and heartaches. And it is healthy and normal to mourn for a season. "To every thing there is a season" (Eccles. 3:1 KJV).

But our human default is to maximize the bad while we minimize all that is still good. This may sound a bit like a lecture, and I don't mean it to be that. It is a pep talk my wife and I have to give each other all the time because life has thrown many hard things at us. It isn't just dealing with the often exhausting complexities of Karin's condition. It is about all the many ways that so much goes wrong in life.

The scary diagnosis of a condition that isn't going to go away. The list of medications. The job that went away. The offer that was so close but didn't pan out. The news from the doctor that surgery is required. The accident. The hospitalization. The huge financial loss through no fault of your own. The terrible boss who insists on signing off on every key decision but then refuses to answer your calls or emails. The death of someone who meant a lot to you.

When life was really rough, we decided to start each day by each mentioning three things we were thankful for. No matter how bad the circumstance we were going through, we forced ourselves to do this exercise.

Dale: "Flowers, the scent of pine trees, and a fresh-picked peach."

Me: "Air-conditioning, indoor plumbing, and Visa cards."

Each day we chose something new. And it really did help shape our attitude for the day.

Go ahead and try it for a week, even if it seems kind of forced or even kind of silly. It can't hurt, and it might help.

# TWENTY

# Patience Is a Virtue

I am often tempted to dress like an Amish person when I go to the grocery store, because it would make it glaringly obvious to the clerks that I should not be expected to use the self-service kiosk. I don't know what it is about me that leads cashiers to believe my transaction would be somehow more efficient or pleasant if I tried to serve myself. But it happens all the time, even when I try to avoid eye contact and slip into the line crammed with senior citizens and those with vision impairments.

I will be in the herd of customers who are lined up and slowly moving forward toward the checkout stands equipped with actual humans who know how to ring up items and strategically place them in bags. And some youthful person, typically sporting a tattoo and nose ring, will tap me on the shoulder and note that there is no waiting in the self-service sector.

"No thanks," I will reply as I offer something between a smile and a grimace.

"But, like, dude. You only have three items and everyone else has a full cart."

"I kind of like slow lines," I will protest weakly as the clerk ignores my wishes, hauls me down the bank of cash registers, and deposits me in front of a touch screen designed by Satan.

The first problem is that the self-checkout system assumes that I am a thief. There is no presumption of innocence. I scan a small package of breath mints and commence fiddling with the plastic grocery bag and a scary computer voice announces, "PLACE THE ITEM IN THE BAG! THE FIRST ITEM IS NOT IN THE BAG!!! PLACE THE ITEM IN THE BAG NOW OR WE WILL OPEN FIRE!!!"

All the other shoppers stare at me as a bulky security guard arrives to monitor my every move.

My next item is a zucchini. It has no UPC code, but I wave it in front of the red scanner beam in the wild hope that somehow the system has been programmed to differentiate between vegetables.

"Oh, you have to enter a code for that one," observes the clerk.

"Well, I meant to memorize all the produce codes but only made it up the rutabagas," I snap.

"It's a 20947," he says.

"How about you walk over here and do it for me since you know what to do and I don't?"

"Well, this is self-service, so that kind of defeats the whole idea."

"Precisely," I reply.

The clerk fails to grasp my point. I sigh and place my last item on the scale. A head of lettuce.

"Code?" I ask Mr. Tattoo.

"You can use the touch screen to pull up an animated representation," he replies.

I slowly turn to stare at him.

"I don't want to touch an animated representation. And I don't want a code. And I don't want a synthesized voice accusing me of shoplifting. And I don't want to have to bring a butter churn to the store so that you people can get the drift that I am a technology dolt who has fond memories of rotary phones. I want to put my items on the counter, hand money to a clerk, and have the clerk put the items in a bag and then I want to leave."

"Then you shouldn't be using self-service," he says.

"Ah, my dear Watson. You're finally catching a clue."

"My name is Jeremy," he replies with a wrinkled brow.

I do not belong in the modern era. But if current technology is challenging for me, it can be overwhelming for an elderly person who is beginning to show signs of dementia.

I often use a gas station that offers a discount if I pay in cash. But this means I can't pay at the pump. I have to enter a tiny mini-mart and hand money to the cashier. And that is how I found myself standing behind Fred and Muriel, who looked like they were both on the sunny side of eighty. They were chatting with Misty, the twentysomething clerk.

Fred: "I tried to use my card at the pump, but it won't work."

Clerk: "That's okay. We can run it from here. What pump are you on?"

Fred: (Long Pause.)

Clerk: "That's okay. I can look at the video monitor. What kind of car are you driving?"

Fred: "Hmmmm . . ."

Muriel: "The blue one."

Clerk: (Looking out the window.) "Okay, it looks like pump three. Just insert your card here." (She pointed at the card reader on the counter.)

Fred swiped the card on the device.

Clerk: "That won't work with that card. You have to insert it. It has a chip."

Fred: "I don't want any chips. I just need gas."

Muriel: "You're doing it wrong, Fred."

Fred: "Then you do it."

Muriel takes over as someone else walks in the door and stands behind me.

Muriel: "So what do I do?"

Fred: "Buy the gas."

Muriel: "I was talking to the young lady."

Clerk: "Just insert the card in the chip reader." (She points to the exact spot to insert the card.)

Muriel inserts it and removes it in one quick motion.

Clerk: "You have to leave it in there until the transaction is approved."

Muriel: "What?"

Fred: "You're doing it wrong, Muriel. Let me take over."

They trade places, in a decidedly unhurried manner, as two more people line up behind me.

Clerk: "Okay, just put the card in that slot and leave it there until I say to remove it."

Fred: "Got it. I used to just slide it on the side. This is different from the way you used to have it."

Clerk: "Yes it is. But the chip is more secure. Okay, it looks like you are using a debit card instead of a credit card, so I need you to enter your PIN."

Fred removes the card from the reader.

Clerk: "No, you have to leave it in there while you use your PIN."

Fred: "I don't have a pen. Can I use yours?"

Muriel: "I have one." (She starts digging through her purse.) More people get in line behind me. Grumbling ensues.

Clerk: "No, your *PIN*. That number you use for your debit card."

Muriel: "I only have a felt tip. Will that work?"

Clerk: "Not a pen. Your *PIN*. It's a number."

Fred: "Can you just do it for me?" (He extends the card toward her.)

Clerk: "Sir, I'm sorry, but I don't know your PIN."

Muriel: "You're doing it wrong, Fred. Let me take over."

They trade places in a leisurely manner. More people get in line.

The clerk asks if they can possibly pay in cash.

Fred: "I left my wallet in the car. I don't like to keep it in my pocket because it hurts my back to sit on it."

Muriel: "He has a terrible back."

Fred: "I just took my card out of my wallet so I could buy the gas. I can go get my wallet."

A groan comes from behind me.

Muriel: "Let me check my purse." (She searches through a large handbag for what feels like an hour before she finds her wallet, opens it, and discovers six dollars and change.)

Fred: "We need to fill up. You used to be able to fill up on five dollars. But not anymore. I used to pay twenty-nine cents a gallon. Those were the days."

Increased grumbling from behind me, and muttered cursing.

Clerk: "Do you have a regular credit card?"

Fred: "A different credit card than the last one?"

Clerk: "Yes."

Fred: "I can get it out of my wallet." He starts for the door, and something bordering on thunder emanates from the crowd that has now reached nine people.

Muriel: "I have a Visa, Fred."

She inserts it and pulls it out in one motion.

Clerk: "No, you need to just put it in and leave it there until I say."

Person in line behind me: "FOR THE LOVE OF GOD, JUST DO IT FOR THEM!"

Clerk: "Store policy is that we have the customer run their own card. I'd get written up!" (She motions at the security camera above her.)

There were a few more false starts as Muriel inserted and removed the card before the transaction was approved, but she finally succeeded in accomplishing the objective. It had taken twelve minutes, and a few of the people behind me were about to need medical treatment for apoplexy. I stepped up to the counter and handed Misty thirty bucks for pump five.

Me: "You were very patient with them. Thank you."

Clerk: "My grandparents are like that, bless their hearts."

Be completely humble and gentle; be patient, bearing with one another in love.

Ephesians 4:2

# TWENTY-ONE

# Double Trouble

"**M**om, did you give ice cream to Dad?"

"Yes. He likes it."

"But he's diabetic."

"I cured it. He also likes cookies."

It is double trouble when both of your parents have dementia at the same time.

Oy vey.

Before she lost her independence, Karin was the primary caregiver for her husband. That would have been fine—had she not been afflicted with Alzheimer's. But we had a year-long struggle to convince Dale's mom, a retired nurse who used to know better, that diabetes is not curable and that giving chocolate chip cookies to her husband was not quite what the doctor had ordered. Her own dementia had her living in utter unreality about Gene's condition.

One day Karin remarked, "Dad really enjoyed driving to the store today."

Dale was aghast.

"Mom, Dad can't drive safely anywhere, even down to the corner, or he could hurt himself or someone else!"

"Your father is an *excellent* driver! By the way, I am heading to Oregon next week."

"Mom, Dad can't be left alone!"

"I'll just stock up on extra cookies for him."

We did what we could to reason with her, but it was fruitless. I decided to get the authorities involved, so I called the office of Adult Protective Services and explained that someone needed to get a handle on the mess.

The person on the other end of the phone listened patiently and then walked me through the reality of the county's caseload, the fact that they had their hands full with seniors who were being abused and neglected, that Dale's parents were blessed to have two people actively engaged and working with them, and that we needed to deal with it.

"You can go to court and get conservatorship if you need to," said the county worker. "But unless they're in immediate danger—as in the house is about to burn down—you and your wife need to handle it. 'Too many cookies' would not even trigger a report. Be strong. Do what you need to do to help them, even if they get mad at you."

Ah. She was right. I was being too much of a wimp.

Dale took a run at it.

"Mom, I was thinking that we could get a visiting nurse to come out a few times a week to check on Dad."

"I am not going to have strangers come into my house to provide medical care," Karin replied.

"But Mom, *you* were a visiting nurse for years. It was *your job* to go into people's homes and provide medical care. *You* were the stranger in other people's homes."

"That's different," Karin replied.

"How?" Dale asked.

"It just is. Now, get your father a bowl of Frosted Flakes. That's his favorite."

Dale tried a new tack.

"Mom, I'd like to bring dinner out to you and Dad tonight. You cooked for me all those years, and I would like to give you a break. How does that sound?"

"That sounds very nice! Thank you!"

So Dale became the personal chef for her mom and dad, and she also picked up "just a few extra groceries" on a regular basis. She made healthy and balanced meals, and stocked up on sugar-free dessert options.

We talked Karin out of her plans to drive to Oregon, and her son called her to reiterate in no uncertain terms that Gene was no longer allowed to drive. For some reason, she listened to her son.

There were several times I seriously suggested to Dale that we go to court to gain the legal authority to take over their lives, but we knew it would poison our relationship with Karin. Ultimately, we decided it made more sense to just amp up our visits and oversight.

It was exhausting, especially for Dale. I could flee to the relative peace of my job, but she was pretty much the caregiver. Karin had other children who could help on occasion, but they lived hundreds of miles away. The burden was mostly ours—mostly Dale's.

I'm sure we missed things—like medications taken at the wrong time or forgotten or tossed out. Things weren't perfect. But they were far better than if Karin and Gene had been left on their own.

Dale's dad lived to a ripe old age even with his diabetes, and it wasn't a complication of diabetes that eventually took his life. So I think we did okay.

If you are in this boat with both parents, you not only have to look out for them as individuals but also try to keep them from accidentally harming each other. There isn't an exact science to this.

When you decide one or both of them can't live in their own place anymore, you might have to take a few runs at getting them dislodged. It is always better if they agree (even though they may later forget that agreement). You may need to invoke the power of attorney form they signed. That form, along with notes from at least two doctors stating that your loved one(s) are no longer competent, will pretty much assure that just about everyone will take your word over theirs (especially once they meet your loved one). It is unlikely the court will ever need to be involved.

A doctor was doing an assessment on Karin and pointed at my wife.

"Do you know who that is?"

"I most certainly do. She's my mother," Karin replied.

"What year is this?" he asked.

"1945," she replied.

He looked at Dale, and his look said, "You get to call the shots."

# TWENTY-TWO

# Moving In, Moving Out, Moving On

Karin and I had this conversation as we helped her pack up some of her belongings in preparation for her first move in forty years.

Karin: "Why are you unplugging my phone?"

Me: "Because we're moving you to your new place, and you'll need your phone."

Karin: "But I still need a phone for when I'm here."

Me: "You won't be coming here, because you're moving."

Karin: "And don't touch the TV, either. I like to watch the news when I'm in the kitchen."

Me: "You can watch TV from your new kitchen."

Karin: "I wish they hadn't taken my license away. I think some busybody turned me in to the department of motor vehicles. Do you know who did it?"

Me: "Hey! I brought some lemon cake! Let's take a break and have some."

Karin: "I've been driving since Eisenhower was president."

Me (using my inside voice): "That might be the problem."

Karin: "What's that thing the doctor said I have?"

Me: "Memory loss."

Karin: "Well, he's wrong. Why is my phone in this box?"

Me: "Because we're moving it to your new home."

Karin: "What will I do for a phone when I'm here?"

Me: "You won't be here."

Karin: "Do you think my doctor told them I'm a bad driver?"

Me: "I think we should have some cake now."

Karin: "That sounds nice! You spoil me."

The Bible tells us that "Love is patient, love is kind" (1 Cor. 13:4).

And love sometimes has to use every trick in the book, especially when your loved one has to move.

Losing her license made Karin even more dependent on us. At that time she was still able to largely function independently, but her home was in a rural area where she couldn't walk to any stores or services. Dale and I were making a twenty-four-mile round trip multiple times per week to bring groceries, help her with tasks, or just to visit with her because she was so isolated. Furthermore, she lived on about six acres of wooded land that needed mowing, weed whacking, branch trimming, and all manner of upkeep she could not possibly perform. The status quo was untenable, but it was *her home* and she did *not* want to move.

So I kept planting the seed.

"You know, Dale and I were thinking that it would be so nice to have you move into town where we could see you more often."

"You see me up here all the time," she replied.

"Yes, but we could see you even more if you lived in Chortling Oaks Center for Chipper and Independent Seniors, that new senior-living place just five minutes from our house. I just happened to pick up a brochure you can look at."

"I'll think about it," she replied—which was her code phrase for *no*.

A week went by and I took another run at it.

"Say, I was just talking with the manager of Chortling Oaks, and she mentioned they have a waiting list. Maybe you should get on it just in case something opens up down the road and you feel like making a move."

"I'm not ready for that kind of decision," she replied.

"And there's no pressure to decide. But if you are on the list, you have the option. You can always say no. If you just sign right here, we can get the paperwork rolling, and there is absolutely no obligation. Dale and I think it is a good idea. But you need to sign up fast, before someone else beats you to it. And did I mention that they have music programs every week and a hymn sing-along time every Friday night?"

"I'll think about it," she said.

Another week passed.

"Hi, Karin. I happened to be near Chortling Oaks, since it's just a convenient five minutes from our home, and I discovered that a bunch of seniors get together each Wednesday and play chair volleyball with a beach ball. They sure were having a blast."

"I've never played that."

"And they watch old Gary Cooper movies in the evening. And they have cake all the time," I said.

"Cake?"

"The place is practically a bakery. Someone is always having a birthday. And there are ladies who just like to bake up a storm. The cake is like manna from heaven, only with more frosting. But you have to be on the list. You can always turn them down, but you have to at least get on the waiting list. It's a hugely popular place, and there could be seniors who are racing down there this very moment to win a spot and get the last piece of cake."

She paused and thought it over.

"Well, I guess it couldn't hurt to just be on the list. As long as I can say no," she said.

She signed on the dotted line.

I waited until I was out the door before I performed a triumphant and highly uncoordinated dance all the way to my car. Any observers would have phoned the paramedics to report a man having a seizure. I burned rubber down to the Chortling Oaks office to turn in the paperwork.

Karin was officially on the waiting list.

No corporate deal maker has ever worked as hard to secure a signature from the other side. No United Nations commission has ever negotiated an agreement that was more daunting to achieve. On my tombstone will be this epitaph: "He got his mother-in-law to sign the paperwork." I think some kind of medal is warranted or even a Nobel Prize or at *least* a really good pizza.

Weeks turned into months as we waited for an opening, and Dale and I took turns making the drive to Karin's home. But we no longer drove daily, and we kept in touch with her a lot by phone. Part of that was just because we were getting burned out by the constant trips, but part of it was strategic.

We wanted her to feel a twinge of need for more social interaction. We hoped she would get tired of being alone.

She kept alternating between "thinking about it" and insisting that she was going to stay in her home and give those DMV people a stern talking-to until they let her resume her rightful standing as a member of the motoring public.

One day, when she seemed a bit pensive, I asked her an important question.

"Karin, what if you had a magic wand? And if you waved it, you would suddenly find yourself living in a nice apartment complex for seniors, and you could visit with neighbors every day. Would you wave it?"

"I don't know if I could afford it," she replied.

"That wasn't the question. The question is about having a magic wand, and whether you would like to have some neighbors to visit with and do things with. Let's suppose the magic wand also included magical loot to pay for it. Doesn't it get kind of old to be stuck out here all on your own with hardly any neighbors? Wouldn't you like to make new friends? Don't you want to be closer to us and your grandkids?"

There was a long pause.

"Well, I think it sounds kind of nice," she admitted.

Church bells pealed, the angels sang, a brass band erupted with "Happy Days Are Here Again," and rejoicing woodland creatures gave each other high fives.

"Well, I have good news. The manager at Chortling Oaks called, and an apartment has opened up. We get to move you next week."

"That soon?"

"Yes. Isn't that great?"

"Well, I'll need to think about this."

"No problem," I said.

It was fine with me if she thought about it—right up to the moment we put her in my car and drove her to her new place and plopped her down on the sofa and made her a cup of tea in her new kitchen. And she could keep thinking about it as she played chair volleyball and went to lunch at the senior center and then had her hair done at the on-site beauty salon that specialized in turning gray hair into a rather unnatural shade of mauve favored by all the other ladies at Chortling Oaks. She could think about it until the second coming of Christ, but there was no way she was going to do anything other than move. We had a signed power of attorney form, and we were prepared to use it.

In the end, she agreed to move on the condition that we would drive her back to her "real home" anytime she wanted to go. It was a small sacrifice to occasionally drive her back up the hill so she could putter around her old homestead for a few hours. And the novelty of it wore off as she adjusted to her new place. She eventually stopped asking to go.

We had done it. We could breathe easier. Sort of. For a while. Until her next move. In seventeen months.

# TWENTY-THREE

# Independent (More or Less) Living

The first year went pretty well for Karin as she settled into life at the Chortling Oaks. And, yes, I am making up the name to avoid a stern letter from a grouchy attorney who has a sense of humor usually associated with prison guards in the old Soviet Union. But it seems like almost all of those assisted-living places have the words *oaks* or *pines* or *whispering* or the maddeningly misused *pointe*.

My friends at the Merriam-Webster company note that the word *pointe* is defined as "a ballet position in which the body is balanced on the extreme tip of the toe."[1]

I have visited a gob of senior-living places, and not one time have I observed a single retiree performing any part of *The Nutcracker*. I have seen lots of moseying and shambling and all manner of leisurely strolling, but precisely zero prancing on tips of toes.

If one is looking for the word to denote "a particular place," the word is *point*! Just plain old *point*. Hey, senior-living facility owners, using the word *pointe* is not a correct use of our mother tongue and certainly not a license to add a premium to your rates, even if your oaks actually *do* whisper. Half your clients have hearing aids. They would probably prefer a few shouting oaks, or at least some pines that would speak up so they could be heard.

(End of rant.)

As I was saying, the first year of independent living went pretty well. Meaning that my mother-in-law was getting along okay on her own, socializing with other folks her age, and generally enjoying life.

Yes, she was getting more forgetful and confused, which we observed more and more when we took her to the grocery store.

"Why are these canned pears in my shopping cart?"

"Hmmmm. I thought you put them there."

"No, I didn't. Someone must have put them here by accident. I don't need them."

"Sure. I'll put them back."

We would meander through the aisles in a decidedly inefficient fashion as she filled up her cart, looked down in surprise at what was there, and had us put half the items back on the shelf. On the plus side, it was kind of like a low impact aerobic workout. Dale and I toned our muscles in our slow jogs through the grocery store.

And, of course, when we were checking out she would have us run back to where we started so we could grab a few cans of pears.

She would forget the name of her neighbors, and often forget she had ever met them.

"Hello. I'm Karin."

"I know. I'm Myrtle and we had muffins together yesterday morning in the community center."

"Well, it's nice to meet you. What's your name?"

"Myrtle!"

"Well, I'm Karin. It's a Swedish name. They have muffins in that big room if you want to join me."

Her memory was clearly slipping, and it made for some awkward conversations, but she was doing well in several other areas. Still cooking. Still using the phone and the laundry facilities. Still taking walks and socializing with understanding friends.

You want to monitor this stage closely, but you also want your loved one to be as independent as possible for as long as possible. Not only is it good for them, but it is the far more affordable option—especially if your loved one is not financially well-off. And a lot of seniors are not financially healthy. A 2016 headline in *Money* proclaimed, "1 in 3 Americans Has Saved $0 for Retirement." The story went on to note that "56% of Americans have less than $10,000 saved for retirement," and "28% of people over 55 have no retirement savings."[2]

Let that sink in. More than a quarter of people who are about a decade from retirement do not have a dime saved up.

The average social security retirement check in 2017 was a smidge over $1,400.00 per month. Yikes. (The average check for men was $1,583.77, while the average check for women totaled $1,231.50.[3] The disparity is due to a complex formula that factors in total years in the workforce, multiplied by stuff that will make your eyes glaze over and have you lunging for the bottle of extra strength Tylenol. Suffice it to say that many women who are currently in their eighties stayed home in the 1950s and 1960s to raise children and cook and clean and get the kids off to school and operate a nonstop chauffer service for their kids while also carving out time to do all the laundry and ironing and vacuuming and waxing the kitchen linoleum and attending PTA meetings and overseeing the homework and bandaging the skinned knees and doing all of the shopping and enormously shaping the next generation—but this means they were not "working" for purposes of calculating their social security benefit. Don't shoot the messenger.)

However, even if a woman was a stay-at-home mom and never worked a day for an employer who gave her a check, she can still typically receive a social security retirement benefit based on her husband's employment (if he worked the required number of years while paying into social security). The Social Security website has all kinds of info on this, and has a pretty good search feature.[4]

Still, even a combined social security retirement income is pretty small. And for many Americans, social security is the totality of their retirement income.

On a brighter note, the real estate website Zillow reports that more than two-thirds of seniors who are seventy-four and older have paid off their mortgages.[5] So that certainly helps, and the home can also be sold if Mom and Dad need to downsize and also need ready cash.

A PBS report a few years ago explained that roughly half of America's private sector workforce is covered by a traditional lifetime pension or a 401(k)-style savings plan. But just about every report on retirement readiness, whether from the Government Accountability Office or a private sector analysis, says that most Americans are not financially prepared for retirement.[6]

*Money* did note that 31 percent of seniors age sixty-five or older have savings balances of $200,000 or more.[7] That sounds like a healthy chunk of change, but Mom or Dad could burn through that in a handful of years in assisted living.

So the goal should be independent living for as long as possible.

Even a market-rate apartment in most cities is far less expensive than assisted living. But Mom or Dad might not have to spring for a market-rate place. There are many independent-living places that are heavily subsidized for seniors with modest incomes. These units are typically going to have a waiting list, so start scouting early. In many cases, the rent is calculated on a sliding scale based on a senior's income and assets.

Don't think "dumpy" when you hear the word "subsidized." Yes, there are sketchy options out there and places to avoid. But many of the subsidized complexes are quite nice. They can charge below market rates because of things like the Low Income Housing Tax Credit (LIHTC) program overseen by the US Department of Housing and Urban Development.

I could get into the mind-numbing details of Section 42 of the Internal Revenue Code, but you don't really need that information unless you have a serious insomnia problem. Suffice it to say, the feds make it worth it to the landlord to offer below market rates, and a couple million affordable apartments have been created nationwide under this program.

(While I am sympathetic to the argument that the federal government could have more efficiently used housing dollars by dropping bails of cash from the backs of C-130 jets flying across the fruited plain, I am simply reporting what is available out there.)

There are also housing subsidies available through other government programs. Many low income folks receive rental assistance via tenant-based housing vouchers from the US Department of Housing and Urban Development (HUD) Section 8 program. You can check out the HUD website, www.hud.gov, for more information, or your city or county housing authority.

But rather than trying to navigate the options on your own, it might be best to chat with someone from your local Area Agency on Aging office. The Older Americans Act of 1965 created a nationwide network of Area Agencies on Aging to serve the senior population. These offices act mostly as providers of information and referrals for services. Do a web search for "Area Agency on Aging in (name of your town, city or county)," and you should be able to connect with a helpful human being who knows what is out there.

Some seniors are in the enviable position of having significant assets. And there are fantastic options for them. Dale and I recently visited an assisted-living and memory-care facility that looked like a high-end resort and featured a professional chef, a spa, a theater with overstuffed reclining seats, a doctor, a physical therapist, a concierge, and a chauffeur. And it was priced accordingly. The memory-care wing had plenty of staff not only to assist the residents but also to engage them in daily activities geared to their abilities. There were music and art programs, and even an aviary for the bird watchers. A staff person offered me a fresh-baked chocolate chip cookie. I tried to check in, but my wife dragged me out of the place.

Most people who are not personally senior partners in a Wall Street investment firm, or named Oprah Winfrey or Warren Buffet, can't afford that kind of living arrangement. So in the next chapter we'll talk about what kind of assisted living is out there for the average person, what it costs, how to fund it, whether to go big or go small, and how to ease your loved one into yet another move.

# TWENTY-FOUR

# A$$isted Living

A fter the ordeal with a police officer (responding to Karin's 911 call) in our room in the wee hours of the morning, we knew we had to look into assisted living. We had learned the hard way that Karin wanders at night. Even if we could put countermeasures in place to keep her from leaving and even if we could unplug the phones and even if we could take the knobs off the stove and plan for all manner of other contingencies, we couldn't prevent her from making noise, knocking on our door, and/or generally making sleep impossible. So we commenced the search.

There is a massive difference between an assisted-living facility and a skilled-nursing facility. They offer very different levels of care, operate under substantially different rules, have different requirements for staff, and charge tremendously different fees.

Think of assisted living as more like a home, and skilled nursing as more like a hospital. The average assisted-living home will not have medical staff. The skilled-nursing facility, as its name implies, has a lot of medical staff. Generally, assisted living is private pay, while skilled nursing involves insurance companies and/or state and federal funding. (There are exceptions, which we will get into later. But this is a general rule.)

You want your loved one to avoid a skilled-nursing facility as long as possible, and hopefully they never need that level of care (or need it only briefly).

An assisted-living home is what the government prefers to call a residential care facility (RCF). They are not medical facilities, although some of the larger places may have some medical staff. But, as the name implies, the goal is to provide care in a more residential atmosphere. Assisted living is about helping your loved one with the activities of daily life when they can't quite manage things on their own. A typical RCF provides a bedroom (usually private, but sometimes shared), regular meals and snacks, guided activities, and twenty-four-hour staff to make sure everyone is okay and that Mom gets pointed back to her bedroom if she gets up in the middle of the night to use the restroom or have a bowl of oatmeal (two of Karin's typical habits). The staff is prepared to redirect anyone who decides it is a nice time to head outside for a 2:00 a.m. stroll or startle a sleeping stranger with a random phone call.

There is typically a base price for an assisted-living place, with additional fees based upon how much additional care is required. (Typically, there is a point system. Costs increase as the number of points push Mom into another category of care. The more pills Mom takes, the more points she accumulates. The more help she needs with daily grooming, the more points are added. Ditto that for feeding and all kinds of other factors. So, as with golf, you want as low a score as possible.)

RCFs are big business in America because we are living longer than ever and coming down with Alzheimer's disease in record numbers.

The Centers for Disease Control and Prevention (CDC) released a great deal of helpful data in its 2010 National Survey of Residential Care Facilities (this is the most recent data set available as this book goes to press). I am going to highlight the key findings and the stuff I found most helpful, but you can visit the CDC website and check out the survey for more information.

"In 2010, residential care facilities (RCFs) totaled 31,100, with 971,900 beds nationwide. . . . *About 4 in 10 RCFs had one or more residents who had some or all of their long-term care services paid by Medicaid.*" (Emphasis added.)[1]

This is the exception to the "private pay" general rule. But don't get your hopes up too soon. Government assistance for assisted living is generally limited to certain kinds of people in specific facilities in limited numbers of beds in certain geographic places. More on this in a bit. The CDC continues:

> Larger RCFs were more likely than small RCFs to be chain-affiliated and to provide occupational therapy, physical therapy, social services counseling, and case management.
>
> Residential care facilities (RCFs)—such as assisted-living facilities and personal care homes—provide housing and supportive services to persons who cannot live independently but generally do not require the skilled level of care provided by nursing homes. RCFs are not federally regulated, and state approaches to RCF regulation vary widely.[2]

Translation: You have to do your homework. You need to visit the facility and spend time observing. When you walked in the door, did it chime? Or was there some kind of access control or alert system so the staff knows someone opened the door?

Does the place look clean and safe? Is there a "home-like" quality to it? Is the staff engaging with the residents? What programs do they offer? What is the staff-to-patient ratio? Check the online reviews for comments of others. Ask trusted medical providers. Ask families who have a loved one there. Be nosy. Unlike nursing homes, RCFs are not subject to strict government oversight. Depending on what state they are in, they might get a visit every several years. Seriously.

Look at the bathrooms. Are there grab bars? Is there a call button/cord? If not, what policy or practice is in place so that staff is available to help (if needed) when the restroom is used?

Falls are one of the primary hazards faced by seniors, whether or not they have dementia. Is the facility free of clutter? Is the carpet or flooring in good shape? Bad flooring can create tripping hazards. Is there anything that will obstruct a cane or walker? Area rugs and throw rugs are basically booby traps for the elderly.

When Karin was living on her own her home was liberally strewn with area rugs, and Dale watched her stumble over the one in the hall.

"Mom, let's get rid of that rug. You almost fell."

"I've had that rug for years and it's fine."

"But Mom, I just watched you almost fall to the floor! What if you had fallen and I wasn't here?"

"I didn't fall, and you worry too much."

Over the next week we observed the malevolent rug trying to bring her down every time she ventured into the hall. She would be shuffling along (precisely the problem) and the rug would lunge at her.

We got her doctor to weigh in.

"Karin, I see this all the time. A senior trips, breaks a hip, ends up bedridden in the hospital, contracts pneumonia, and the next thing you know the family is planning a memorial service. I would like you to get rid of all the throw rugs."

"I'll think about it."

We thought about it too—and whisked the rugs away from her home.

How is the lighting in the assisted-living home? You don't want it either too dim or too bright. You don't want Mom tripping over a chair because a glaring lightbulb distracted her.

Do the chairs have armrests so Mom can stabilize herself when sitting down or getting up?

Ask to see the protocol for administering medications. There should be a rigorous and crystal-clear method for the dispensing of meds. The staff should be aware of every medication Mom or Dad takes, and that includes over-the-counter stuff. If you are taking Mom out for the day, staff should know about it and send medications with you with written instructions on when (and how) the meds need to be taken.

While it should be a given that each RCF has twenty-four-hour staff, make sure that the home or facility requires that there is "awake staff." In the overwhelming number of cases, that will be true. But verify it so you don't do business with a place that lets a staff person sleep on the night shift. You are paying good money for this care, and your loved one deserves attentive staff at all hours.

The CDC notes that the types of services offered at RCFs vary by facility size.

Nearly all RCFs provided basic health monitoring (96%), incontinence care (93%), social and recreational activities within the facility (99%), special diets (93%), and personal laundry services (99%). Small RCFs were less likely to provide social services counseling (24%) and case management (51%) than larger RCFs. Medium RCFs were also less likely to provide case management (57%) than larger RCFs. Extra large RCFs were most likely (91%) and medium RCFs were least likely (73%) to offer transportation to medical or dental appointments.[3]

There are pros and cons to each size and type of facility. The small places are often just slightly modified homes nestled in a residential neighborhood. There are just a handful of residents, and the home can have kind of a nice "family" feel to it. So they really feel like a home. But these places often lack the kind of regular outings and services provided by the bigger places. It is a trade-off.

The place we chose for Karin was a six-bedroom house in a residential area. It looked like a regular home, because it pretty much *was* a regular home. And that is one of the things we liked about it. There were six residents, and the living room had enough recliners for all of them.

There was a fenced backyard with a large lawn, shaded porch areas, and carefully manicured plants and flowers. As expected, there was twenty-four-hour "awake staff" to assist and interact with residents, do laundry, cook, clean, and administer medications per doctor's orders.

The staff—all ladies—were great. They understood dementia and were skilled in redirecting and de-escalating.

"I need my car *right now*, and I need to go find my mother!"

"Sure. We can do that in just a bit, but I have all these towels to fold. I wonder if you could help me for a few minutes? I'm just so behind on my chores."

"I'm happy to help! You should have asked sooner."

"You're so sweet!"

Karin was placed in one of three neighboring houses. Two were side-by-side with the other behind them, so they formed a triangle. The original fencing had been reconfigured so there was one large yard. Residents were assigned a house based on where they were in the progression of the disease. House one was for zero/mild dementia, house two was for moderate, and house three was for late moderate/advanced. Karin was placed in house two.

Wow. I just noticed how simple I made that sound. "Karin was placed in house two." It's just six words. I can also use just six words, concisely and accurately, to say that "NASA landed men on the moon." But the short phrase does not convey the epic amount of planning and effort.

So let me back up and explain how we made it happen, and help walk you through some strategies that may help as you plan to move your loved one.

The decision was made at about 2:30 a.m., when the police officer made one last comment before heading back to his car. I previously explained that the officer had responded to a 911 call Karin placed from our home when she could not figure out where she was, or why her husband was missing.

The officer looked at us and said, "When she starts calling us in the middle of the night, it's time."

We knew exactly what he meant, and we knew he was right. She could not go back to her apartment. Independence was not possible. We also realized that she was simply too much for us to handle.

While we had done some preliminary looking and interviewing with assisted-living operations, we thought we would have more time to decide.

Karin, Dale, and I were all wide awake and talked for hours after the officer left.

Karin could acknowledge that she had indeed been in our house many times, and that she had gotten confused, and that something was awry with her mind.

"I think I need to be checked out," she said at last.

We gave her a hug, unplugged the phones, got her back to bed, and I called a local hospital that had just opened a geriatric mental health wing. I explained what had happened, and they advised me to bring her to the hospital in the morning.

"She'll need to be admitted to the ER first," the nurse informed me. "They need to get her checked out and rule out other conditions, such as a bladder infection. Something as simple as that can create confusion. If they clear her medically, we can evaluate her for admission to the geropsych unit."

We got back into bed after 4:00 a.m. and tried to get a few hours of sleep.

Morning came too soon. We got up and made breakfast. Had extra coffee. But we didn't make a beeline for the hospital. There was an important detour.

We had made early morning arrangements to bring Karin to the assisted-living home we had selected for her. First, the management needed to meet her to make sure our description of her (sweet-but-befuddled former nurse) matched the reality. Because not every home is going to take every potential resident. If someone hits, bites, yells, tries to escape, or has other difficult behaviors or needs, they are going to be harder to place. And they are going to cost a lot more than a cheerful and compliant resident who is reasonably mobile. So we walked in the door with Karin and met the owner.

"Hello, I'm Mike. It's nice to meet you," he said, shaking her hand.

"Well, nice to meet you! My name is Karin, not Karen. Everyone gets it wrong because it is Swedish," she explained.

"Really?" he said. "I'm half Swedish and half Norwegian."

"The Swedish part is better," she said, and laughed.

Then I chimed in.

"Karin knows how to count to ten in Swedish."

On cue, she rattled off, "En, två, tre, fyra, fem, sex, sju, åtta, nio, tio."

"Wow," Mike said.

Karin smiled.

Mike took her on a tour of the home and introduced her to the staff and to other residents. While she was visiting with another sweet little old lady, Mike pulled Dale and me aside.

"She will fit in very well. Come back later, and we'll get the paperwork done and get a deposit."

As we wrapped up the visit I asked Karin what she thought of the home.

"It's very nice," she said.

"Mom, could you see yourself living here?" Dale asked.

Without a pause, Karin replied, "I think that could be very nice."

Then we drove to the hospital. Karin was in the emergency room for a few hours as a battery of tests were run.

"This seems like far more than is necessary. I'm not having a heart attack, and I'm not bleeding," she groused.

And she was kind of right. It was a bit of overkill. But it was required by protocol.

As we suspected, it wasn't something simple like an infection or a vitamin deficiency. So she was wheeled to the third floor and became the second patient to be admitted to the brand-new geriatric mental health wing.

She loved it. She had spent her entire working life as a nurse and missed it deeply when she retired. Suddenly, she was back on the floor of a hospital. And the other nurses on duty had eighteen empty rooms and were eager to get rolling as they waited for more admissions.

It was like attending a nurse reunion. They fussed over Karin, made sure she had everything she needed, listened to her stories of being a nurse, and generally treated her like royalty.

But within a short amount of time, Karin was asking, "Now, about all these children who are wandering around the halls. Shouldn't they be in school? Where are their parents? Are they our patients? If so, I need to see charts."

The staff seamlessly went into professional mode.

"Carol will take care of the children, won't you, Carol?"

Nurse Carol nodded.

"In the meantime, I want to show you one of our new rooms. I think you'll be impressed with the lovely view of the mountains," said Nurse Jan.

In a short amount of time, Karin's mind convinced her that she was on staff, having been hired to help the younger nurses learn the ropes. But she was also there to take a few classes.

The "classes" consisted of various memory tests, group therapy (it was a very tiny group), and putting together a puzzle. She stayed five days, and at the end, the attending doctor explained that she didn't have a treatable mental illness. She simply had Alzheimer's disease. But we felt good about going the extra mile just to make sure that her original diagnosis was correct. I believe in second opinions.

Plus, having her in the hospital bought us time so we could bring her bed, clothes, and a few special belongings to the Festive Acres Assisted-Living Home and get her room set up. We hung favorite family photos and art on the walls. We also used the time to give notice at her apartment, move many things to our garage, and sell off or donate excess furniture and household items.

Shrinking down a lifetime of accumulated stuff was a step of its own. And it was hard on Dale, even when the items wouldn't seem to have sentimental value.

Because it wasn't just any old sofa—it was her mom's. And it wasn't just any old recliner—it was her mom's favorite chair. It wasn't just a simple maple dinette set with white chairs—it was the place where Karin served us lemon cake and talked about how much she loved her view and the day she saw a deer walk by. We were boxing up or selling off the last physical vestiges of Dale's mom's independence.

It was hard to see the apartment empty. It had been transformed from a home into a sterile void. We had worked so hard to get her there and to tastefully arrange it for the first day she moved in. We have a photo of her standing in the kitchen, smiling, eyes twinkling, and showing off her new digs.

She had enjoyed nice neighbors, like the charming woman from Jamaica who wore flamboyant colors and spoke with the most lovely island accent. There was the tiny little lady who rode in a motorized wheelchair decked out with American flags and a red, white, and blue string of lights, and who (in good weather) never missed being outside to watch the sunset. And, of course, there was the woman formerly known as Esther who used to ride with us to church.

It was hard on Dale to lock the apartment door for the last time, because that click of the lock meant that the independent chapter of Karin's life was over, and the "assisted" part was beginning.

I gave her a hug.

Karin wasn't quite ready to leave when we came to get her discharged from the hospital.

"I like it here. Everyone is so friendly. And I don't think my shift is over."

The nurses gathered to wish her well.

Karin, who by now had been promoted to charge nurse, reminded them to keep on top of their charting. And then we drove to Festive Acres.

There are different ways to handle the handoff. Mike's preferred system was to have people bring their loved one over for lunch and quietly slip away while the residents were busy visiting over chicken and dumplings. He thinks the adjustment is easier if you aren't hovering nearby.

Others suggest staying for that first meal. A lot of it will depend on the level of confusion your loved one is feeling.

If Mom or Dad is aware they are moving into a new place, they may have some anxiety. (Think about your first day at a new school or a new job.) Mom or Dad might worry about fitting in. And if they were resistant to the move, they might be mad that it is happening.

Keep in mind that the staff is practiced in doing this, and your loved one is going to be receiving a lot of attention to make the transition as smooth as possible. The staff may try to pair your loved one with a compatible resident—a buddy system. It is amazing what can happen when a couple of seniors become new friends.

Karin was soon holding hands with another sweet lady. It was like they were old friends having a reunion. And that might have been what they were thinking. Works for us!

Staff can also, at least initially, try to keep your loved one away from Mr. Grumpy, who is still pretty sharp and is in assisted living mostly for physical problems that are just too much for his spouse to handle anymore.

"Welcome to the stalag. Watch out for Frau Müller. She'll call the guards if you try to bust out of here."

Don't panic or second-guess your decision if Mom makes it clear she isn't pleased to be here. It can take time for her to adjust. If it is a good home with caring staff, you're doing the right thing.

For the first few days Karin asked why she was there and when she was going home. There is no perfect way to handle that question. We never said, "This is your new home." We told her at first (and somewhat truthfully) that her doctor wanted her to be here for a while (with "a while" defined as "for as long as possible").

That satisfied her for a bit. Sometimes she would get agitated because she imagined an urgent situation that required her immediate attention.

"I left the dog in the car!"

The first time that happened, Dale assured her mom that a friend had been up at the house and let the dog out.

"That makes no sense!" Karin replied. "Why would she be at my house, and how would she get my keys?"

So that failed.

When the same issue came up again, Dale told her mom, "I checked with Dad, and he let the dog out."

"I'm so glad you told me!" Karin replied. "You have no idea what a burden that takes off me."

Dale has basically become a really practiced improv artist.

Likewise, staff can often think of something that works. But if it is an ongoing problem, and Dad is aware he isn't at home and objects to being where he is, you just have to keep trying new angles and hope you find one that works. I wish I had a better suggestion.

Visit often. If Mom is mobile, take her on outings. Encourage her to participate in organized events facilitated by the home. Karin has been on patio boat excursions at a lovely local lake. Sometimes a singing group will pop in to serenade the residents. Craft projects are a nice diversion and a chance to do something social. Check out the activities calendar (and follow up to make sure Mom is encouraged to participate if she is able).

And keep her moving as much as possible on a daily basis.

A nurse who works with seniors told me, "Avoid a wheelchair unless it is absolutely necessary. Walkers yes, wheelchairs no. Muscles can atrophy amazingly fast. If you took

Arnold Schwarzenegger at the peak of his fitness and put him in a bed for twenty-eight days, I guarantee you that he wouldn't be able to get up and walk. Keep her moving. Don't let her default to just sitting or sleeping all day."

The larger RCFs are more likely to have staff with the specific task of keeping your loved one physically and mentally engaged. And larger facilities have more residents to choose from to match seniors who have similar abilities and interests. The smaller places may have just one person on at a time, and that staff member might be tasked with taking care of everything that crops up. In between checking on residents, assisting them with the restroom, cleaning, and cooking, they are also supposed to have an activity going to keep the residents as engaged as possible. It is a tall order. Some staff are total rock stars and really do pull this off. But you want to be around enough to observe. A sleeping resident is an easy resident, but that is not what the doctor ordered. It isn't what she needs.

Mom doesn't need to be bored. Her mind still works; it just has a lot of deficits. If she can do activities and enjoy walks in nature, make sure it is happening. In bad weather, walk with her someplace enclosed.

And keep her laughing, if possible. I will deliberately say absurd things to see if I can get a laugh out of her. It is also my own way to test her cognitive skills.

I will bring out a boxed coconut cream pie and say, "You will never believe what I whipped up today."

"You're right, I won't," she replies.

"I had to personally lasso the coconuts as they tried to scamper away. I barely caught enough to make the pie," I continue.

She shakes her head and laughs.

"I don't believe a word he says. Well, at least on this subject."

She reaches over to squeeze my wife's hand.

"I'm so glad to have you as my little sister."

"Me too," Dale replies.

# TWENTY-FIVE

# Hospice Is Not a Bad Word

Someone pulled us aside for a conversation.

"I don't want to worry you, and I'm not saying that the time has come, but I think we need to discuss hospice care."

We were blindsided by the words. Hospice is the kind of service you get at the very end of life. Karin had been doing well according to her baseline abilities, and no doctor had hinted that she was in her last months, so we were simply taken aback by the very word *hospice*.

"Is there something we need to know?" Dale asked.

"Just level with us," I added.

"No, I'm not saying she is at that point. I'm not a doctor. I just want you to have it on your radar screen so you know what is available to you when the time comes. You want to know what hospice offers before you need it."

He was right.

So I researched it.

So here it is.

Both Medicare and Medicaid can cover hospice services, which can be rendered in a home, hospital, assisted-living or skilled-nursing facility, or a hospice facility. Hospice care is an intense level of service—often revolving around pain management—when a doctor determines that someone is likely to live six months or less. But hospice is so much more than pain management.

From the get-go, let me emphasize that hospice care should not be equated with medically induced death. There are some states that have legalized physician-assisted suicide. I live in one of those states. But I am morally opposed to that, and it is emphatically not what I am talking about.

Hospice is also not giving up on Mom or agreeing to substandard care because the end is near. Indeed, hospice contains a wide array of services, including 24/7 care if it is needed. Medical services and supplies can still be provided. But because the premise of hospice care is that the patient has less than six months to live, that twenty-four-hour access to a hospice team member is more about comfort and pain management, as opposed to heroic medical intervention and mad dashes to the hospital.

Although medical professionals are involved in hospice, at its very core the hospice movement is a volunteer effort by incredibly thoughtful and dedicated people. The volunteers play a huge role. They are more than willing to go shopping and run errands while you focus on your loved one. In the absence of or in conjunction with family, the hospice volunteers provide companionship and friendship. They have all been trained and provide a great bedside manner. They will perform small acts of service such as writing letters for Mom or Dad or reading to them or putting on some favorite music.

Yes, they even do dishes. And laundry. And babysitting. Pretty much whatever is needed, these folks are there to do it. Because they really do care, and they find it deeply gratifying. Jesus once said it is more blessed to give than to receive, and hospice volunteers find that to be true in their own lives.

When that hard day comes, and your loved one leaves this world, the hospice volunteers are there for the family. They are a shoulder to cry on, and they can be a blessing. Your doctor or area hospital will likely be able to give you information on local hospice options. And there are many options.

I have found hospice ministries that are explicitly Christian, funded by donations, and offered at no charge to the patient. Hospice programs that are not explicitly religious will almost certainly accommodate the religious preferences of the patient. And there are generic hospice chaplains that will offer foggy "spiritual" words that might not remotely match the beliefs of your loved one. So understand what is being offered, and use discernment about who is offering spiritual support. If Mom is a lifelong Baptist, she won't derive comfort from someone who starts talking about karma or becoming one with the universe.

> When I come to die
> When I come to die
> Oh, when I come to die
> Give me Jesus
> From an old spiritual,
> author unknown

# TWENTY-SIX

# They Call Me a Wanderer

So here is the short version about the day I was carjacked: I was at a stoplight when a total stranger walked up to my car, flung open the passenger door, took a seat, and demanded that I drive him where he wanted to go.

What would you do? Resist? Comply? Hope someone noticed and called the police? Experience a hygienic lapse that requires a change of pants?

I didn't try any karate moves, since my abductor was on the sunny side of eighty years old and looked like he was about to pass out.

So here is the long version: I live in a city that is known for its blistering hot summers. Our town has officially logged mercury at the 118-degree mark, which I think is slightly higher than the suggested temperature for baking muffins. Unless you have been in that kind of heat, you can't imagine just how appalling it is. It is miserable in the shade, downright painful in the sun, and about twenty degrees worse if you're surrounded by blacktop. It is akin to strolling through the Sahara, only with fewer Bedouins and camels and a lot more testy drivers.

I had been stopped at a long light on one of those wickedly hot days. On the corner stood an excessively senior citizen in a Panama hat and leaning on a cane. And at that moment, he decided he couldn't take it anymore. So he walked to my car, opened the door, and got in.

"Take me home," he said, gulping in the air that blasted from the air conditioner vents. Now, if he had been sixty years younger and covered with scary tattoos, I would have scampered out of the driver's seat faster than you can say "fugitive felon." But I didn't believe the octogenarian posed a mortal threat to my person.

He had no water. He was utterly unprepared for the heat. So I got him hydrated and asked him where he lived. And when he told me I was stunned, because it was several miles away and up a steep hill in an area known for numerous apartment complexes . . . and most of the large assisted-living facilities in town.

At that time, Alzheimer's just wasn't on my radar screen. So I dropped him off where he said he lived, and then I went back to my own errand. I can only hope he really did live there and that he got safely back into his own place. I shudder when I think just how clueless I was that day.

It was several years later, on yet another scorching day, and in the midst of Karin's dementia issues, when I saw an old man making his way down the sidewalk of a busy street near our neighborhood. I was on my way to a store and got about halfway there when a little warning bell went off in my head. So I turned around and drove back to check on him.

He was in about the same spot, but now walking in the opposite direction. No rational person would be taking a pleasure stroll on that kind of day and on that kind of street.

I pulled up next to him and rolled down my window.

"Do you need some help, sir?" I asked.

"No. Just heading to the senior center," he replied.

"It's Sunday, sir. The senior center is closed."

He looked perplexed.

"How about if I give you a ride home? It's kind of hot today," I ventured.

"That sounds good," he said, and got in the passenger seat.

I gave him water (no one leaves without water in the car during summer in my town, any more than an astronaut would leave his oxygen back on terra firma).

"Where's home?" I asked.

"It's, um, up there a bit," he said, pointing vaguely north.

I headed north.

"Just tell me when to turn," I said.

And thus began our long and scenic outing. If anyone had been watching from an airplane, they would have assumed the driver was utterly lost, or perhaps trying to throw off a surveillance vehicle. My passenger didn't have a wallet or any form of identification, so I had no address to shoot for.

"This looks like it," he said for the fifteenth time on the fifteenth street when I finally pulled over and prepared to phone the police.

But as I reached for my phone, he pulled a phone from his pocket.

Lifesaver!

"Is there someone you can call?" I asked.

"I live with my daughter," he said.

"Do you know how to call her?" I asked.

He flipped open the red Jitterbug phone (a model designed for easy use by senior citizens) and punched a couple of buttons.

It rang a few times and then I could hear the female voice on the exceptionally loud phone.

"Hi, Dad. How *crackle* you today?"

"I want to go home. I'm in the car with the man."

"Dad? Are you with Michael? Hand the *crackle crackle* to Michael."

He handed the phone to me.

"Hello. My name is Dave, and I'm with your dad. He was walking in my neighborhood, and . . ."

"MICHAEL *crackle* HIM OUT ON HIS OWN???!!! I'LL *crackle* HIM!!!"

"If you can just give me an address, I'll take him home."

"*Crackle crackle* . . . a THOUSAND TIMES that Daddy can never *crackle crackle* . . ."

"How about if I . . ."

". . . CANNOT BELIEVE . . . *crackle* . . ."

"I can bring him to you," I said, deeply grateful not to be Michael.

"I am in Portland at a *crackle*, and the cell service is absolutely *crackle crackle crackle*."

And then we lost the connection. I hit the scroll button and found that her number was the only one stored in the list. Great.

"It's just over there," the old man said, pointing and looking eager.

I decided to give it one more try before heading to the police station. I turned onto a street and saw a guy my age striding briskly down the sidewalk, desperately glancing from side to side. I pulled up next to him and rolled down the window.

"Excuse me, would you happen to know this—"

"Harold! Oh, thank God!" he exclaimed as a wave of relief washed over him.

"I found him on Shasta View," I said.

"All I did was go use the restroom. Seriously! He was out of my sight for five stinking minutes and vanished into thin air. How can someone that old move that fast? Oh, thank God that Gwen doesn't know about this!"

I didn't have the heart to break the news that Gwen would likely be expressing her opinion of his caregiver skills once she got back home. I hope Michael will regain at least some of his hearing when she is finished.

A wandering person with dementia is, obviously, a serious problem (especially for Michael). Memory-care facilities have alarmed doors, fenced outdoor areas, and awake staff twenty-four hours a day. But if a person with a form of dementia is staying in your home, you don't have the luxury of full-time staff. With enough coffee you can manage to pull an all-nighter, but the novelty of that wears off pretty fast. And, like Michael, when you gotta go, you gotta go.

Here are a few suggestions on minimizing the risk of harm if a loved one does wander off.

First, and easiest, get a bracelet for them. It should have their name, the best number to reach you, and notation of "Alzheimer's" or "impaired memory" engraved on it. A bracelet that can't be unclasped is better than a necklace they can promptly toss in the trash. You can have a bracelet made for you at an engraving shop.

The bracelet won't prevent wandering, but it sure helps whoever finds your loved one (unless you are in Portland in a bad cell area, in which case you might want to have two phone numbers available).

The next step is to make sure your neighbors know the score. Have a recent photo available. If your loved one has a wallet, print up a card explaining that he has Alzheimer's and include a number to call. The wallet might get lost or thrown away (Harold had no wallet when I picked him up), but it is still a good idea. You can also stick a card in their pocket. Have it laminated, and it will be almost indestructible.

Sometimes you can kind of figure out why they are wandering, and sometimes it is a mystery. Many wanderers want the familiarity of home, and they are determined to get back to it. They may just say, "I'm going home!"

Your home doesn't feel like their home. Depending on how cognizant your loved one may be, you may be able to reassure them that they are in the right place, you really would love to have them stay, and this is their new home. If they feel calmed and welcomed, they may be less prone to wander. But get used to reminding them. A lot.

But if they are pacing, agitated, and fixated on escaping, you have a major challenge on your hands. You can try distracting them by having them "help" you with something like folding the laundry, sweeping, dusting, putting a simple puzzle together, reading a story to you—whatever might work. You can also offer to take a walk with them. A trip around the block might do the trick.

You will need to get the right hardware to lock the doors if Mom or Dad is dead set on leaving. You can place a couple of those flip locks, one high and one low, on the doors. Unlocking one or both of them may be too complex for the wanderer to overcome. If those gadgets don't work, try something else. Childproof devices can double as Alzheimer's proof devices to keep your loved one out of the kitchen and bathroom cabinets. Plastic, kid-proof doorknob covers can be one more level of complexity that will stump your wanderer. You can also put chimes on the doors. Make sure you install hardware that keeps the windows from opening all the way.

If your loved one wanders at night, you really have to amp up the precautions. We found out the hard way that Karin is up at all hours of the night. That is how we ended up with a cop in our bedroom. She can get by on an astonishingly small amount of sleep.

Folks with dementia can still often turn on a stove, but lose the ability to remember to turn off the flame. Can you see a potential problem here—one that involves fire trucks and lots of yelling and smoke and lengthy explanations to the insurance company, or worse?

If you are dealing with a night wanderer, you might need to invest in an electronic floor pad next to her bed that alerts you when her feet touch the floor. Or a similar gizmo that wakes you if she opens her door or window. There are a lot of products on the market, and a lot of them are inexpensive and effective. The more fundamental issue is whether you are ever getting a decent night's sleep. If you aren't, and everyone is groggy and crabby and starting to hate life, you probably need to consider a different living situation for your loved one. The good news is that there are some really fine options out there. The bad news, as we have seen, is that the costs can be a big challenge unless you work at Fort Knox—and they start allowing the employees to have free samples.

# TWENTY-SEVEN

# Resentment, Fear, and Other Hazards of Caregiving

You never imagined being a caregiver. You didn't plan on Alzheimer's being a daily part of your life. There was no way you could have foreseen all the demands on your time, all the hundreds of details that had to be handled, the odd behaviors you would have to cope with, and the bizarre fibs you would have to tell.

It can lead to burnout. Exhaustion. Resentment. Depression.

While your mind tells you that your dad didn't choose this disease, your emotions can scream, "How can he not know where the bathroom is when he uses it every single day? I can't take this anymore!"

Emotions can be stronger than rational thought.

I think of myself as a pretty analytical kind of guy, but I routinely prove that emotion can overwhelm my intellect.

Case in point: many years ago I found myself more than six hundred feet in the air standing on a thin band of steel that was ready to snap. Why had I ever agreed to do this? What would it feel like to fall? Would there be something left to bury?

The thin strand of metal swayed. I sucked in my breath and waited for the massive *twang* of metal snapping, followed by the violent jolt that would hurl me to my shrieking demise.

"Hey, Dad! I think we can make it rock more if we run back and forth!" exclaimed my son Mark.

"This is so cool!" chimed in my other son Brad.

I could have really used some Depends at that moment.

We were inside the St. Louis Gateway Arch, the tallest stainless steel monument in the world. And the wind was making it sway. Engineers will explain that the arch's legs are sturdy equilateral triangles with stainless steel skin covering carbon steel walls that are reinforced with concrete from ground level to three hundred feet. The guys with pocket protectors will also note that the legs are buried sixty feet deep in more than twenty thousand tons of concrete. And that the arch is *not* going to fall over. But I'm not an engineer, and I was petrified, so it sounded like a bunch of hoity-toity mumbo jumbo. I *knew* I was going to die.

That was more than two decades ago. And when I checked the news today, the arch was still standing.

My emotions that day were powerful and at odds with reality.

Emotions are stronger than rational thought.

Ask anyone who is terrified of spiders or has a phobia of cats. These are not rational feelings. But they are real, and strong.

Here are some feelings that can hit someone who cares for a loved one with Alzheimer's:

*I can't do this anymore.* This is a marker of exhaustion. This person is worn out by the huge demands of living day-to-day with this disease.

*I am going to go off the deep end, or drop dead, and then there won't be anyone else to take care of him.* There can be enormous anxiety about the future. If you are plan A—and there is no plan B—caregiving can create a lot of fear. You can also feel trapped or like you are drowning.

*I'm too tired to go out with friends. It's easier to just stay with Mom.* It can be tempting to withdraw. But a caregiver can't afford to just have their world reduced to nonstop caregiver duties. Even if it takes effort to get someone else to take over for a day or just an evening, that effort is vital. You have to have a break. There are adult daycare places, and people can also be hired to come into the home. Totally worth it.

*I give up.* You may be depressed. If you have no energy, have lost interest in things you used to enjoy, and just can't manage to pull things together, you really need to see a professional. Counseling, even medication, may be necessary. You don't necessarily have to be sad to be depressed.

The Centers for Disease Control and Prevention notes that "Depression is more than just feeling down or having a bad day. When a sad mood lasts for a long time and interferes with normal, everyday functioning, you may be depressed. Symptoms of depression include:

- Feeling sad or anxious often or all the time
- Not wanting to do activities that used to be fun
- Feeling irritable, easily frustrated, or restless
- Having trouble falling asleep or staying asleep
- Waking up too early or sleeping too much
- Eating more or less than usual or having no appetite
- Experiencing aches, pains, headaches, or stomach problems that do not improve with treatment
- Having trouble concentrating, remembering details, or making decisions
- Feeling tired, even after sleeping well
- Feeling guilty, worthless, or helpless
- Thinking about suicide or hurting yourself."[1]

This is serious, and you should not just try to "power through it."

But even if you don't wrestle with depression, caregiving can result in other negative thoughts and feelings.

*If she does that one more time, I'm going to snap.* The combination of exhaustion and the nature of the disease can make a caregiver feel anger. This is not a good place to be. Beating yourself up or lecturing yourself to "snap out of it" is not going to overcome the emotion. You need some help, and you need a break.

*No one understands what I'm going through.* You really are inhabiting an unusual world, and most of the people you know do not understand it. But that does not mean they cannot help you. Confide in a friend. Go out for coffee. Get away for a weekend. All of these powerful emotions are canaries in the coal mine. They are signaling that something needs to change.

*What do you mean I missed the appointment? What appointment?* Forgetfulness and getting overwhelmed are not uncommon for caregivers.

*I don't remember what it's like to laugh, or to enjoy life.* That statement, and any of the aforementioned statements, are causes for concern. Having a tough day is expected and normal. But if these thoughts are consistently running through your head, you need help. You need to make your own physical and mental health a priority, or there is no way you are going to make it for the long haul.

I used to tell Dale, "This is a marathon, not a sprint." But I think that is the wrong analogy. This is actually a relay race, and the baton needs to get handed off. A marathon lasts 26.2 miles, not years on end. So don't think of yourself as *the* runner. Think of yourself as a runner on a team.

"But Dave," you might say, "we don't have the money or the people. It's all on me."

I would urge you to take the time to really examine whether or not that is true. Even if you bear the primary burden, look into the programs that are out there. Don't discount friends, other family members, and the church. Spend Mom's or

Dad's resources. And if they don't have resources, don't discount the public resources available. Hey, you've been paying taxes all your life. It is okay to get some of them back in this time of need. As we have seen, Medicaid is a live option when Mom's or Dad's resources have been expended.

Some people have a default position of thinking they don't need help, and, even if they come to the conclusion that they do need it, they don't want to seek help. But this is not a sign of strength. It is actually a sign of insecurity—not that I am ever one of those people.

A couple years ago I was in Hawaii and leaped off a small rock ledge for a plunge into the Pacific Ocean. I spent some time snorkeling among festively colored fish while simultaneously looking out for mutant electric eels that would happily kill me.

I read about electric eels when I was a kid and have harbored a pathological fear of them ever since. My irrational dread isn't mitigated by the fact that the electric eel is not an eel at all, but a species of freshwater fish that lives in South America, which is quite a distance away from Hawaii. The mere fact that there exists an aquatic creature capable of generating a lively eight-hundred-volt jolt is enough to give me the jitters in any body of water that is not contained in a bathtub.

When it came time to clamber out of the ocean, I found that the rocky point from which I had entered was quite a bit higher than I remembered. The tide had begun to go out. I reached high and made repeated efforts to grasp the ledge but was having difficulty as wave after wave slammed me into the rocks and then sucked me away just as I was managing a bit of a grip.

Suddenly, a hand reached down to me. I didn't know the guy and felt a bit embarrassed, so I gave it another go on my own and was knocked around by another wave.

"Trust me, it'll be easier this way," he said.

I took his hand, and he hauled me up.

Whether you are floundering in the ocean or in life, when someone offers you a hand, you should take it.

# TWENTY-EIGHT

# Don't Bail Out Now

You know it is coming, and you try to sort of brace for it, but nothing makes it easier.

"She asked me my name," Dale said.

"Honey, I am so sorry," I replied.

And then I babbled on about how this was probably just a temporary thing, and that Karin might have just been tired, and that she would remember again, and this was likely just part of the ebb and flow of the disease, and let me try to fix this because that's what men are prone to do when the best thing we can do is probably just give her a hug and tell her we love her.

Because even though Karin did recognize Dale on future occasions, nothing removes the sting of that first time your mom looks at you and honestly doesn't have a clue who you are.

It is, indeed, a hard thing.

We have noticed a disheartening reaction from people who will abandon a lifelong relationship when someone develops an impaired memory. They sometimes actually say something like, "Well, if they don't know who I am, there's no use visiting them."

These are the same people who would make ongoing trips to the hospital room of someone with cancer or who was involved in a bad accident. But they make an exception for dementia.

Memo to those people: this isn't about you.

Your friend is still your friend, and your family member is still your family member, even in an impaired state. Even if they don't recognize you and can't recall all those memories you used to share. Besides, they may enjoy meeting new people. You can be the new friend that keeps surprising them with how much you have in common.

"You brought blueberry pie! That's my favorite! What a coincidence!"

If you can still bring them a moment of companionship, it is worth your time. If you can hold their hand or read them a story or a favorite psalm or show them some funny videos on your phone, do it. This is about your friend or loved one in a time of need. This isn't about your feeling "uncomfortable" and therefore running away. This is about sacrifice. About giving. About doing something for someone else, even when your emotions are urging you to flee.

Too often we reduce "giving" to cutting a check. I'm all in favor of sending loot to churches and other good causes, but sometimes "giving" has to be in a different form.

This is about being the courageous soldier who doesn't leave his buddy on the battlefield.

Listen, I totally get it. I get the exhaustion of trying to come up with something to talk about when the person you are chatting with doesn't know whether you are her uncle, her doctor, or the UPS driver. I get hating the atmosphere of the hospital or the other institutional setting. Dale and I completely get the grief of watching this slow-motion train wreck play out over the years.

Today, when I asked Karin whether her name was of Swedish origin, she looked puzzled and replied, "I'm not sure about that."

Having a Swedish name is something that has been a big deal to her for more than eighty years. She has always delighted in pointing out that her name was not Karen. And it just poofed into thin air. These kinds of incremental losses break our hearts on an ongoing basis.

We totally get the pain of watching someone suffer and not being able to make it stop. And we understand that life still has to go on, and the bills have to get paid and the lawn needs to be mowed and the laundry isn't going to wash itself and on and on and on.

But today, as Karin was in bed at a rehab hospital, we were able to make her laugh. Several times.

And she probably forgot it about thirty seconds after we left. But we had that moment, and it lifted her spirits, and it was important to her and I believe it was important to God. He is totally into even very small gestures. "And whoever in the name of a disciple gives to one of these little ones even a cup of cold water to drink, truly I say to you, he shall not lose his reward" (Matt. 10:42 NASB).

There are future divine rewards for being a kind and compassionate person for Christ's sake. Bringing flowers earns you future credit in heaven. But there is also the reward *right now* of becoming a more generous, thoughtful person. It is way too easy for me to be self-absorbed. Acts of self-sacrifice and kindness are antidotes to being self-centered. This is Jesus stuff, if you think about it.

That Alzheimer's sufferer is making you a better human being, if you allow it.

# TWENTY-NINE

# A Life More Real Than This One

Here's a helpful kitchen tip: If you're making a salad and run out of tomatoes, you can substitute by cutting small wedges from an old Goodyear tire. While the tire is a bit on the chewy side, it has more flavor than the average store-bought tomato.

I never thought I liked tomatoes—until I had a real one from a local garden. That's when I discovered there is a galaxy of difference between garden-fresh heirloom tomatoes and the fake, reddish orbs sold in typical grocery stores. To be fair to your local produce manager, it isn't that he actually wants to provide you with bland imitation fruit. The problem is that commercial farmers cannot successfully transport the kind of wonderfully sweet, deeply red, juicy, messy, tender, bursting-with-flavor tomato that God invented.

An authentic tomato is the type you need to gently pluck warm from the vine, cradle in your hand, carry into your house (preferably on a pillow), and eat the same day, when it is at the height of ripe perfection. If you loaded these kinds of tomatoes into a cargo bin and stuck them on a truck, they would be tomato juice by the time you drove two blocks. So industrious agricultural researchers have created hybrid versions that look a lot like the real deal but are sturdy enough to remain intact at the bottom of a truckload of boulders. These engineered tomatoes are so hardy that they will remain unfazed even if you beat them with a crowbar (which is what they deserve).

So I grow my own. Last summer my backyard was home to six robust plants, lovingly staked, watered, mulched, weeded, fertilized, and heavily guarded by a stout guy called Louie the Fist.

There is such a vast difference between my tomatoes and the store variety that I feel truly sorry for people who have based their opinion on the sham version. They have no idea just how good the real deal is.

Just like I rejected the bogus version of tomatoes, many people have rejected the dull, tasteless, phony version of heaven. I think one of the devil's biggest and most successful con jobs has been the caricature of heaven—a monotonous place of strumming instruments—that appeals to a small percentage of elderly members of the Methodist Ladies Knitting Circle.

Nonsense.

The best earth has to offer is a pale imitation of what awaits us in heaven. Seen the Grand Canyon? That will be a snoozer compared to the sights in glory. The best food you have ever tasted will seem like swill compared to the tastes of heaven. The best experiences you have ever had on earth, or wish you'd had (and I'm including the best fishing, the best vacation, the best sports victory, and the best human experience you have ever enjoyed) will pale in contrast to the incomparable experiences of heaven.

The place that awaits us above won't be a step down from earth. It won't be fishing, vacation resort, sports, or whatever you utterly enjoy now. It will be something unfathomably, outrageously better. Jesus will bowl us over with himself and the array of stuff he has planned for our enjoyment. Think a real tomato is great? Just wait until you bite into heaven!

The very concept of heaven, of an eternal life after death, looms larger when you love someone who could soon be stepping from this world into the next.

It was a Friday morning, and I was about a month away from the deadline for this book when we got a call that Karin had taken a fall. A doctor was called in to the assisted-living home and ordered X-rays, which revealed Karin had broken her wrist and her pelvis. An ambulance was ordered to get her to the hospital. We arrived at the ER a few moments after she was wheeled into a room.

Mercifully, the ER was not swamped that day, and a medical team was quickly making Karin comfortable, administering pain meds, fashioning a splint for her wrist, and completing the paperwork to admit her. Eight different people played some kind of role, and Karin pointed out to most of them that she was a nurse.

"Your oxygen is at eighty-four," noted a nurse as she prepared to administer the gas.

"Goodness, that *is* low," Karin replied.

The nurse inserted the small tubes into Karin's nostrils, and Karin promptly removed them.

"That tickles, and I don't like it," she said.

"But we need to get your oxygen levels up," the nurse replied, putting the tubes back in.

"I don't like it," Karin said, removing the tubes again.

Dale tried taking over the tube insertion duties.

Karin refused.

"What happens if someone has low oxygen?" I asked the nurse.

"Well, to start with, she's going to get more confused," she said. Great. Just what Karin needs. "She needs sufficient oxygen, or it's going to harm her brain," the nurse continued.

Thus began a series of varied attempts to get more oxygen into Karin's lungs. We tried putting the tubes in her mouth and having her breathe through her mouth. We tried changing the angle of the tubes in her nose. Dale tried just holding the tubes under her nose. We tried reinserting the tubes after Karin was conked out on pain medication.

We had varying degrees of success for short amounts of time, but Karin would ultimately end up removing the tubes. It was exhausting and exasperating to fight that battle.

"Mom, you were a nurse. You know that you need to get your oxygen levels up."

"I'm still a nurse. And I don't like how it feels, and I'm not going to have that in my nose."

In the end, we had to settle for whatever little victories we could achieve for short periods of time.

"I've never been to this place. What's it called?" Karin asked.

Dale gave her the name of the hospital, not feeling the need to point out that it had been a landmark in town for years, that Karin used to know it, and had been a patient there only two years ago.

"It's new," Dale said.

"Why is this cast on my arm?" Karin asked.

"You had a fall and broke your wrist."

"Really? This is the first I've heard of it."

X-rays were reviewed, a CAT scan was performed, and a doctor summed up the situation.

"We set the wrist, but the fractured pelvis is inoperable. It will have to heal with time. But, of course, the difficulty is that she'll get weaker from being bedridden. It would be hard enough for a younger and stronger person to walk again after the weeks and even months she'll be recovering. We just can't project what the future will hold for her."

The doctor went on to explain that Karin would remain in the hospital for the next few days.

"Today is Friday, and a skilled-nursing facility doesn't admit on the weekends. So she's going to be here at least three days," the doctor said.

(Reminder: a minimum three-day hospital stay triggers Medicare coverage in a skilled-nursing facility or rehabilitation hospital.)

Four days later, we had Karin admitted to a rehab place. They started physical therapy three times a day, seven days a week. Every day, and multiple times per day, Karin wondered what had happened to her, and why she was there.

It was slow going, but there was progress. And Karin was enjoying meeting lots of new people.

During lunch in the common dining room, a woman introduced Karin to another patient and said, "This is my mother-in-law."

Karin replied, "She's my mother-in-law too!"

Dale heroically bit her lip to not laugh.

Rehab is a critical time, and Dale was at the facility pretty much daily. We were only too aware of the common pattern of a fall resulting in a lot of bedrest, which leads to atrophy, which leads to even less mobility, which can create a downward spiral into pneumonia.

I asked a nurse about the connection between inactivity and pneumonia.

"Your lungs want to fill up with fluid," she replied. "But for a healthy person, you ward that off by moving and deep breathing."

The nurse went on to note that immobility, coupled with the fact that hospitals are full of germs no matter how fanatically the janitorial staff does their job, means the welcome mat is out for pneumonia. It can kill you.

The physical therapy, coupled with time, eventually got Karin standing (with supports) and moving again (ever so slowly).

But even if she makes enough progress to leave the rehab hospital and return to assisted living, we know that mortality awaits. Not just for her, but for all of humanity.

Many decades ago, Karin settled the issue of where she would go after she died. If you have not done so, it is time to have that conversation with God.

For God did not send his Son into the world to condemn the world, but to save the world through him.

John 3:17

# THIRTY

# A Few Final Thoughts

No, you didn't sign up for this. But it's a big part of your life now. You can't wish it away or pray it away. And because you're a decent person, you don't run away, even though there is sometimes a powerful impulse to do precisely that. We all feel it.

If the person with Alzheimer's is your spouse, this is definitely in the "for better or for worse" category. But really, in any relationship that matters, you are always there in good times and in bad. "For better or for worse" comes with the territory of loving somebody.

To love another means to risk your heart. It means giving more than you ever thought you could. It means desperate prayers for strength and grace, because you just feel so wrung out by it all.

But prayers for grace reach the ears of God, and the answer is always yes.

The heartache comes in a hundred different forms. Alzheimer's is one way. But there is also:

The prodigal son, who has walked away from you and into a life of drugs and deception.

The daughter who married the creep, even though you tried to warn her, and now she seems so trapped.

The spouse who struggles with debilitating depression.

The way the recession ruined so much of what you had built over so many years.

The epic hurricane that took out your neighborhood.

The war that claimed your grandson.

And

    on

      it

        goes.

We all suffer in our own ways, but we all indeed suffer. But it will end. It is limited by time.

In the meantime, in ways that you can't even comprehend, the way you respond to the tragedies of life is shaping your soul.

I have seen people become amazing, heroic, and selfless. I have watched people become awful, immature, and selfish. So much rides on what we do in response to what hits us.

God is watching. Angels are looking on. Heaven is cheering you on, even though you can't hear the applause that breaks out every time you do the right thing, the hard thing, the thing you did not think you had it in you to do.

God is not going to forget a single heroic and sacrificial thing you have done. And he is storing up lavish rewards beyond your comprehension as you serve him by serving one of his suffering children.

Jesus: "I was sick and you looked after me."

Us: "Uh, when was that?"

"The King will reply, 'Truly I tell you, whatever you did for one of the least of these brothers and sisters of mine, you did for me'" (Matt. 25: 34–40).

Jesus takes this personally.

I hope that this little book has provided some helpful information, pointed you in the right direction, and allowed you to smile—and maybe even laugh out loud—when that was exactly what you needed. I hope it has also reminded you that more is going on here than just a disease process. Much more. So much more, your daily life is of cosmic significance. Someday you will see just how big a deal this all was, and it will take your breath away.

So keep on keeping on. Don't go it alone. Lean on those friends, avail yourself of every resource, worship God, walk the dog (even if you don't have one), breathe deeply, have that piece of pie, and take care of yourself in the middle of all this.

But do press on, one day at a time, leaning heavily on the God who loves you beyond your wildest dreams.

> I would have despaired unless I had believed that I
>     would see the goodness of the Lord
> In the land of the living.
> Wait for the Lord;
> Be strong and let your heart take courage;
> Yes, wait for the Lord.
>
> Psalm 27:13–14 (NASB)

# NOTES

## Chapter 1 Sweet Little Lies

1. "Dementia," World Health Organization, last modified December 2017, http://www.who.int/mediacentre/factsheets/fs362/en/.

## Chapter 5 This Is Not Normal

1. "Alzheimer's Disease Information Page," National Institute of Neurological Disorders and Stroke, last modified May 23, 2017, https://www.ninds.nih.gov/Disorders/All-Disorders/Alzheimers-Disease-Information-Page.

2. "Vascular Dementia," Alzheimer's & Dementia, Alzheimer's Association, accessed April 2, 2018, https://www.alz.org/dementia/vascular-dementia-symptoms.asp.

3. "About Dementia with Lewy Bodies," Dementia with Lewy Bodies, Alz.org, Alzheimer's Association, accessed April 2, 2018, https://www.alz.org/dementia/dementia-with-lewy-bodies-symptoms.asp.

4. Michael D. Geschwind, Aissa Haman, and Bruce L. Miller, "Rapidly Progressive Dementia," author manuscript, National Center for Biotechnology Information, National Institutes of Health, July 6, 2009, https://www.ncbi.nlm.nih.gov/pmc/articles/PMC2706263/.

5. "What Is Dementia?" Alzheimer's Association, accessed April 2, 2018, http://www.alz.org/what-is-dementia.asp.

6. "Alzheimer's Stages: How the Disease Progresses," Mayo Clinic, last modified November 24, 2015, https://www.mayoclinic.org/diseases-conditions/alzheimers-disease/in-depth/alzheimers-stages/art-20048448.

7. "Alzheimer's Disease Fact Sheet," National Institute on Aging, last reviewed August 17, 2016, https://www.nia.nih.gov/health/alzheimers-disease-fact-sheet.

8. Anja Schlabon et al., "Frequency and Consequences of Violence and Aggression Towards Employees in the German Healthcare and Welfare System: A Cross-Sectional Study," *BMJ Open* 2, no. 5 (October 2012): 1, http://bmjopen.bmj.com/content/2/5/e001420.

## Chapter 7 I'm Feeling Fine

1. "State-by-State Advance Directive Forms," Everplans, accessed April 2, 2018, https://www.everplans.com/articles/state-by-state-advance-directive-forms.

2. Kuldeep N. Yadav et al., "Approximately One in Three US Adults Completes Any Type of Advance Directive for End-Of-Life Care," *Health Affairs* 36, no. 7 (July 2017): 1, https://www.healthaffairs.org/doi/abs/10.1377/hlthaff.2017.0175.

3. Barbara L. Kass-Bartelmes and Ronda Hughes, "Advance Care Planning, Preferences for Care at the End of Life" *Research in Action*, no. 12 (March 2003): 2, https://archive.ahrq.gov/research/findings/factsheets/aging/endliferia/endria.html.

## Chapter 10 Dr. Finster's Miracle Dementia-B-Gone Elixir

1. "Basics of Alzheimer's Disease and Dementia," Alzheimer's Disease & Related Dementias, National Institute on Aging, accessed April 2, 2018, https://www.nia.nih.gov/alzheimers/topics/alzheimers-basics.

2. "Mrs. Winslow's Soothing Syrup," The Wood Library-Museum, accessed April 2, 2018, https://www.woodlibrarymuseum.org/museum/item/529/mrs.-winslow's-soothing-syrup.

3. Nathan Birch, "The 10 Most Insane Medical Practices in History," *Cracked*, November 20, 2007, http://www.cracked.com/article_15669_the-10-most-insane-medical-practices-in-history.html.

## Chapter 13 Some Can and Do; Some Can't and Shouldn't

1. "Stanford Study Focuses on Effects of Family Caregiving for Patients with Alzheimers Disease and Dementia," *Stanford Medicine News Center*, May 2, 2002, https://med.stanford.edu/news/all-news/2002/05/stanford-study-focuses-on-effects-of-family-caregiving-for-patients-with-alzheimers-disease-dementia.html.

## Chapter 16 Paying for All This

1. Genworth, *Genworth 2015 Cost of Care Survey*, March 2015, https://www.genworth.com/dam/Americas/US/PDFs/Consumer/corporate/130568_040115_gnw.pdf.

2. Christine Caffrey et al., "Residents Living in Residential Care Facilities: United States, 2010," *NCHS Data Brief* 91, (April 2012): 2, https://www.cdc.gov/nchs/products/databriefs/db91.htm.

3. "Life Insurance & Disability Insurance Proceeds," IRS, last modified December 6, 2017, https://www.irs.gov/faqs/interest-dividends-other-types-of-income/life-insurance-disability-insurance-proceeds/life-insurance-disability-insurance-proceeds.

4. AARP has a concise and informative article worth checking out at http://www.aarp.org/relationships/caregiving/info-01-2010/women_life_settlement.html.

5. Elderlife Financial Services (website), accessed April 2, 2018, https://elderlifefinancial.com/.

6. "FHA Reverse Mortgages (HECMs) for Seniors," HUD.gov, accessed April 15, 2018, https://www.hud.gov/program_offices/housing/sfh/hecm/hecmabou.

7. *Reverse Mortgages: Product Complexity and Consumer Protection Issues Underscore Need for Improved Controls over Counseling for Borrowers: Testimony before the Special Committee on Aging*, U.S. Senate (2009) (statement of Mathew J. Scirè, Direct Financial Markets and Community Investment), https://www.gao.gov/new.items/d09812t.pdf.

8. Use the website www.va.gov or call 1-844-MyVA311 (1-844-698-2311) to get routed to the right place.

9. "Assisted Living and Home Health Care," Vets.gov, last modified June 28, 2017, https://www.vets.gov/health-care/about-va-health-care/assisted-living-and-home-health-care/.

10. "History—VA History," U.S. Department of Veterans Affairs, last modified March 8, 2018, https://www.va.gov/about_va/vahistory.asp.

## Chapter 17 Medicare and Medicaid—How They Will and Won't Help

1. Gary Smith et al., *Understanding Medicaid Home and Community Services: A Primer*, October 1, 2000, https://aspe.hhs.gov/basic-report/understanding-medicaid-home-and-community-services-primer.

2. "Costs in the Coverage Gap," Medicare.gov, accessed April 2, 2018, https://www.medicare.gov/part-d/costs/coverage-gap/part-d-coverage-gap.html.

3. "Your Medicare Coverage," Medicare.gov, accessed April 2, 2018, https://www.medicare.gov/coverage/skilled-nursing-facility-care.html.

4. "Medicaid for Millionaires," *Wall Street Journal*, February 24, 2005, Review & Outlook, https://www.wsj.com/articles/SB110920966481062758.

5. "Nursing Home Costs: Nursing Home Costs by State," Skilled-NursingFacilities.org, accessed April 2, 2018, https://www.skillednurs ingfacilities.org/resources/nursing-home-costs/.

6. "Medi-Cal Eligibility and Covered California—Frequently Asked Questions," California Department of Health Care Services, accessed April 2, 2018, http://www.dhcs.ca.gov/services/medi-cal/eligibility/Pages /Medi-CalFAQs2014a.aspx.

7. "Code of Federal Regulations," Social Security, April 2, 2018, https://www.ssa.gov/OP_Home/cfr20/416/416-1210.htm.

**Chapter 18  Are You Smoking Something?**

1. Antonio Currais et al., "Amyloid Proteotoxicity Initiates an Inflammatory Response Blocked by Cannabinoids," *Nature Partner Journals: Aging and Mechanisms of Disease* 2 (2016): accessed April 2, 2018, https://www.nature.com/articles/npjamd201612.

2. Susan Scutti, CNN.com, "Medical Marijuana Has Potential as Alzheimer's Treatment, Study Says," July 25, 2016, http://www.cnn.com/20 16/07/25/health/alzheimers-medical-marijuana/index.html.

3. Scutti, "Medical Marijuana."

4. "FDA and Marijuana," U.S. Food & Drug Administration, last modified February 28, 2017, https://www.fda.gov/NewsEvents/Public HealthFocus/ucm421163.htm.

5. P. Newhouse et al., "Nicotine Treatment of Mild Cognitive Impairment," *Neurology* 78, no. 2 (January 2012): 91–101, http://n.neurology .org/content/78/2/91.short.

6. "Nicotine May Slow Progression to Alzheimer's Disease," Georgetown University, January 9, 2012, News, https://www.georgetown.edu /news/slowing-down-of-alzheimers-may-involve-nicotine.html.

**Chapter 23  Independent (More or Less) Living**

1. *Merriam-Webster*, s.v. "pointe," last modified April 1, 2018, https:// www.merriam-webster.com/dictionary/pointe.

2. Elyssa Kirkham, "1 in 3 Americans Has Saved $0 for Retirement," *Money*, Time, March 14, 2016, http://time.com/money/4258451/retire ment-savings-survey/.

3. Todd Campbell, "How Big Is the Average Person's Social Security Check?" The Motley Fool, August 30, 2017, https://www.fool.com/retire ment/2017/08/30/how-big-is-the-average-persons-social-security-che.aspx.

4. "Benefits for Your Spouse," Benefits Planner: Retirement, Social Security, accessed April 2, 2018, https://www.ssa.gov/planners/retire /applying6.html.

5. Nalina Varanasi, "Free and Clear American Homeowners," Zillow Research, January 9, 2013, https://www.zillow.com/research/free-and-clear-american-mortgages-3681/.

6. "Can You Afford to Retire?" Frontline, PBS, last modified May 16, 2006, https://www.pbs.org/wgbh/pages/frontline/retirement/need/.

7. Kirkham, "1 in 3 Americans."

### Chapter 24 A$$isted Living

1. Eunice Park-Lee et al., "Residential Care Facilities: A Key Sector in the Spectrum of Long-Term Care Providers in the United States," *NCHS Data Brief* 78 (December 2011): 1, https://www.cdc.gov/nchs/products/databriefs/db78.htm.

2. Park-Lee et al., "Residential Care Facilities," 1.

3. Park-Lee et al., "Residential Care Facilities," 4.

### Chapter 27 Resentment, Fear, and Other Hazards of Caregiving

1. "Mental Health Conditions: Depression and Anxiety," Centers for Disease Control and Prevention, last modified January 23, 2017, https://www.cdc.gov/tobacco/campaign/tips/diseases/depression-anxiety.html.

**Dave Meurer** is an award-winning author and talented humor writer whose columns and articles are featured in major publications such as *Focus on the Family*, *New Man*, *In Touch*, *Marriage Partnership*, and *HomeLife*. He is a graduate of California State University at Chico and earned a dual degree in political science and information and communication studies. Dave is the dedicated husband to Dale, father of two boys, and a caregiver to his mother-in-law who has been diagnosed with Alzheimer's disease. He lives in northern California where he serves as community liaison at Klamath River Renewal Corporation, undertaking the largest dam removal and river restoration project in United States history.

PROVEN TECHNIQUES FOR
## IMPROVING AND
## PROTECTING YOUR
# MEMORY

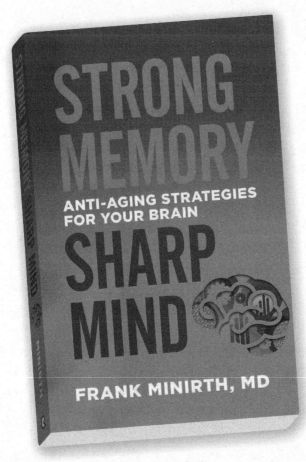

Revell
*a division of Baker Publishing Group*
www.RevellBooks.com

Available wherever books and ebooks are sold.

# Be the First to Hear about Other New Books from REVELL!

Sign up for announcements about new and upcoming titles at

## RevellBooks.com/SignUp

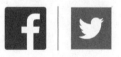

Don't miss out on our great reads!

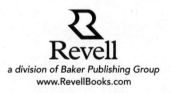

a division of Baker Publishing Group
www.RevellBooks.com

DISCARDED BY
CAPITAL AREA DISTRICT LIBRARIES